Executive Skills in Children and Adolescents

The Guilford Practical Intervention in the Schools Series

Kenneth W. Merrell, Series Editor

Executive Skills in Children and Adolescents

A Practical Guide to Assessment and Intervention

PEG DAWSON
RICHARD GUARE

THE GUILFORD PRESS
New York   London

© 2004 The Guilford Press
A Division of Guilford Publications, Inc.
72 Spring Street, New York, NY 10012
www.guilford.com

Printed in Canada

This book is printed on acid-free paper.

Last digit is print number: 9 8 7 6 5

Library of Congress Cataloging-in-Publication Data
Dawson, Peg.
    Executive skills in children and adolescents : a practical guide to assessment and intervention /
Peg Dawson, Richard Guare.
        p. cm. — (The Guilford practical intervention in the schools series)
    Includes bibliographical references and index.
    ISBN 1-57230-928-8 (pbk.: alk. paper)
    1. Executive ability in children.   2. Executive ability in adolescence.   3. Self-management
(Psychology) for teenagers.   4. Self-management (Psychology) for children.   I. Guare, Richard.
II. Title.   III. Series.
    BF723.E93D39 2004
    155.4′ 13—dc22
                                                                                    2003015732

About the Authors

Peg Dawson, EdD, is a licensed clinical school psychologist with an undergraduate degree from Oberlin College and a doctorate from the University of Virginia. She is currently a staff psychologist at the Center for Learning and Attention Disorders, an agency within Seacoast Mental Health Center in Portsmouth, New Hampshire. Dr. Dawson has over 25 years of experience working in the fields of education and psychology, with a specialization in assessment of children and adults with learning and attention disorders. In addition to working in schools and mental health centers in New Hampshire and Maine, she has also taught in the Education Department at the University of New Hampshire at both the graduate and undergraduate levels. Active in professional associations, Dr. Dawson has been president of the New Hampshire Association of School Psychologists, the National Association of School Psychologists, and the International School Psychology Association. She has also served as the newsletter editor for the National Association of School Psychologists, and has published many journal articles and book chapters on topics related to educational policy and practices and learning and attention disorders. In addition to *Executive Skills in Children and Adolescents,* Dr. Dawson and her colleague Richard Guare have written a manual on coaching students with attention disorders.

Richard Guare, PhD, is a neuropsychologist and currently serves as Director of the Center for Learning and Attention Disorders in Portsmouth, New Hampshire. Dr. Guare received his doctorate in school/child psychology from the University of Virginia and completed a postdoctoral fellowship in neuropsychology at Children's Hospital/Harvard Medical School. He has served as a consultant to a number of brain injury programs in New England, and has presented and published research and clinical work on acquired brain injury and attention disorders. In addition, Dr. Guare has been Adjunct Professor of Communication Disorders at the University of New Hampshire and teaches courses in child neuropsychology at the University of Southern Maine.

Preface

Executive function is a neuropsychological concept referring to the cognitive processes required to plan and direct activities, including task initiation and follow-through, working memory, sustained attention, performance monitoring, inhibition of impulses, and goal-directed persistence. While the groundwork for development of these skills occurs before birth, we believe they develop gradually and in a clear progression through the first two decades of life. But from the moment that children begin to interact with their environment, adults have expectations for how they will use executive skills to negotiate many of the demands of childhood—from the self-regulation of behavior required to act responsibly to the planning and initiation skills required to complete chores and homework. Parents and teachers expect children to use executive skills even though they may little understand what these skills are and how they impact behavior and school performance.

Our first introduction to executive skills came through our work with children and teenagers who had sustained traumatic brain injuries. Problems involving planning and organization, time management, and memory, as well as weaknesses with inhibition and regulation of emotions, have long described a significant component of traumatic brain injury. Executive skills have also assumed an increasingly important role in the explanation of attention-deficit/hyperactivity disorder (ADHD). While our introduction to these skills originally came in our work with these populations, we have seen a growing number of youngsters who seem to struggle in school because of weaknesses in executive skills even when they do not meet the diagnostic criteria for ADHD or another disorder. We believe that these students will benefit from interventions designed to improve executive functioning. To do so, however, requires an understanding of what executive skills are, how they develop in children, and how they impact school performance. We have written this book to shed light on these important cognitive processes so that parents and teachers can better help children hone these skills for the purpose of achieving long-term independence—the ultimate desirable outcome of childhood.

While this book is written primarily for school psychologists and other educational professionals such as social workers, guidance counselors, and special educators, whose

vii

job it is to work with youngsters whose executive skills may be impaired, we also believe that the book will be of interest to clinical psychologists who see these children in private practice or a therapeutic setting, as well as regular education teachers and parents whose job it is to help children apply executive skills to the demands of the classroom and tasks of daily living.

OVERVIEW OF CONTENTS

Chapter 1 defines what is meant by executive skills and provides a list of 11 separate skills that we have included in the construct of executive functioning. This chapter also includes a description of how these skills develop from infancy on and provides a list of the kinds of developmental tasks for which executive skills are required and the ages at which we expect children to perform such tasks.

Chapter 2 describes the variety of techniques that can be employed to assess executive functioning in children and adolescents, including the use of clinical interviews, behavior rating scales, behavioral observations, and formal test instruments. The chapter concludes with a case example designed to illustrate the integration of these various techniques into a single assessment.

Chapter 3 outlines a process for linking assessment to intervention, beginning with the identification of specific skill weaknesses and their behavioral manifestations and leading to the development of multimodal intervention strategies based on the behaviors of concern. The process is illustrated using the same case example detailed in Chapter 2.

Chapter 4 provides both a broad overview of intervention strategies as well as specific strategies to address each of the 11 specific executive functions we have identified. The intervention strategies include environmental modifications, incentive systems to motivate children to use executive skills they may already possess, and instructional procedures to teach skills they have not yet acquired. Each skill is illustrated with a vignette to show how the strategies may be applied in real-life situations.

Chapter 5 provides a more detailed description of "coaching," an umbrella strategy that we believe has wide application for helping students acquire executive skills.

After completing the first five chapters, readers will undoubtedly understand that helping children develop executive skills can be a long-term and labor-intensive process, depending on the severity of the skill deficit. Chapter 6 provides an overview of classroom-wide interventions that can enable teachers to impact skill development in whole classes of students, thereby reducing the need for individually designed interventions.

Finally, Chapter 7 discusses executive skills as they may appear in special populations such as children with acquired brain injury, ADHD, autism spectrum disorders, and sleep disorders and sleep deprivation. The chapter also provides some guidance as to how to approach "complicated cases" such as students with multiple learning or behavior problems. The conclusion of this chapter includes some final "caveats" that readers should keep in mind as they attempt to use the strategies presented in the book with the populations of children with whom they may work.

ACKNOWLEDGMENTS

Publication of this volume has been a long time in coming. It follows years of clinical practice in which we refined our understanding of executive skills and how they impact the development of the children with whom we have worked.

For their help in bringing this work to fruition, we would like to thank our editors at The Guilford Press, including Senior Editor Chris Jennison and Series Editor Kenneth W. Merrell, who kept us moving toward our end goal and who offered suggestions that enabled us to produce a final version that was measurably superior to our first efforts. Their insightful comments prodded us to think more clearly about both how we conceptualize our work and how we design interventions.

We would also like to thank Seacoast Mental Health Center, both for understanding that children with learning and attention problems are as much in need of service as children with psychological and emotional problems and for supporting our efforts to meet the needs of this population.

Finally, we would like to thank the countless children, parents, and teachers over the years who have contributed to our understanding of the role executive functions play in human development. Included in this group are our own children (Aaron and Isaac Dawson and Colin and Shannon Guare), who have taught us firsthand how executive skills develop over time and have convinced us that it *is* possible to intervene successfully to enhance executive skill development.

PEG DAWSON
RICHARD GUARE

Contents

1

Overview of Executive Skills

Human beings have a built-in capacity to meet challenges and accomplish goals through the use of high-level cognitive functions called executive skills. These are the skills that help us to decide what activities or tasks we will pay attention to and which ones we will choose to do (Hart & Jacobs, 1993). Executive skills allow us to organize our behavior over time and override immediate demands in favor of longer-term goals. Through the use of these skills we can plan and organize activities, sustain attention, and persist to complete a task. Executive skills enable us to manage our emotions and monitor our thoughts in order to work more efficiently and effectively. Simply stated, these skills help us to regulate our behavior.

In a broad sense, executive skills help us to do this in two ways. One way involves the use of certain thinking skills to select and achieve goals or to develop problem solutions. These skills include the following:

- *Planning*—The ability to create a roadmap to reach a goal or to complete a task. It also involves being able to make decisions about what's important to focus on and what's not important.
- *Organization*—The ability to arrange or place things according to a system.
- *Time management*—The capacity to estimate how much time one has, how to allocate it, and how to stay within time limits and deadlines. It also involves a sense that time is important.
- *Working memory* —The ability to hold information in mind while performing complex tasks. It incorporates the ability to draw on past learning or experience to apply to the situation at hand or to project problem-solving strategies into the future.
- *Metacognition*—The ability to stand back and take a bird's-eye view of oneself in a situation. It is an ability to observe how you problem solve. It also includes self-monitoring and self-evaluative skills (e.g., asking yourself, "How am I doing?" or "How did I do?").

1

These skills, then, help us to create a picture of a goal, a path to that goal, and the resources we will need along the way. They also help us to remember the picture even though the goal may be far away and other events come along to occupy our attention and take up space in our memory. But in order to reach the goal we need to use some other executive skills in a second way to guide or modify our behavior as we move along the path. These include the following:

- *Response inhibition*—The capacity to think before you act. This ability to resist the urge to say or do something allows us the time to evaluate a situation and how our behavior might impact it.
- *Self-regulation of affect*—The ability to manage emotions in order to achieve goals, complete tasks, or control and direct behavior.
- *Task initiation*—The ability to begin a task without undue procrastination, in a timely fashion.
- *Flexibility*—The ability to revise plans in the face of obstacles, setbacks, new information, or mistakes. It involves adaptability to changing conditions.
- *Goal-directed persistence*—The capacity or drive to follow through to the completion of a goal and not be put off by other demands or competing interests.

When do we need these skills? For the most part, we don't need them to manage our day-to-day habits and routines. We do need them when we face a new challenge or resolve to pursue a goal.

DEVELOPMENTAL TRENDS

As we noted above, executive skills are built-in. But while they are built-in, executive skills obviously are not developed at birth or for some time after that. We see their beginnings in the infant and toddler and even more of them in the 5-year-old. But even in the 15-year-old, we sometimes marvel at the lack of planning, time management, or especially inhibition. So these skills, which are at the heart of self-regulation or self-control, begin to develop in early infancy and continue to develop well into adolescence. If we can understand how these skills improve through childhood, we can begin to understand how much control children exercise over themselves at different ages. This information in turn can help us as adults to know how much support and structure to provide as children develop.

EXECUTIVE SKILLS AND BRAIN DEVELOPMENT

Before we consider the developmental sequence, however, we need to look briefly at the way executive skills relate to the brain and brain development. At birth, the child's brain weighs about 400 grams. By late adolescence this has increased to about 1,400 grams (Kolb

& Wishaw, 1990), or from 13 ounces to a little less than 3 pounds. A number of changes in the brain account for this significant growth. Rapid generation of nerve cells (neurons) and their supporting cells (neuroglia) takes place in the brain. These cells are the building blocks of the nervous system. In order for nerve cells to "talk" with each other, they develop branches that allow them to send and receive information from other cells. The growth of these branches, which are called axons and dendrites, is especially rapid during the infant and toddler periods. Finally, in order for such "conversations" between the neurons to be efficient, the branches that carry these conversations (as nerve signals) need to be insulated. The insulation, which increases the speed of nerve signals, is provided by a substance known as myelin that forms a fatty sheath around the axon. The process, called myelination, begins in the earliest stages of development and continues well into adolescence.

Thus, there is a parallel between development of the brain and development of the child's ability to act, think, and feel. This parallel is especially important in understanding how executive skills develop and what areas of the brain are most critical for these skills. Researchers now generally agree that frontal brain systems (the frontal/prefrontal cortex, along with connections to adjacent areas) make up the neurological base for executive skills. Figure 1.1 depicts the human brain with the approximate location of major functions, including executive skills in the prefrontal cortex.

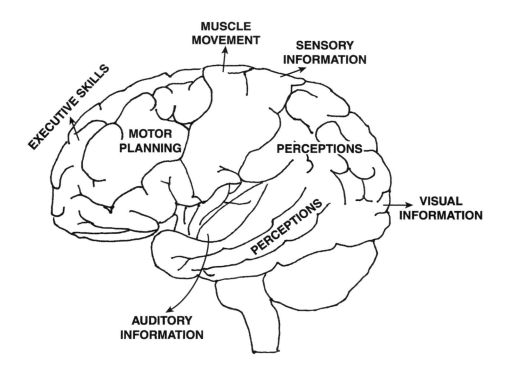

FIGURE 1.1. The human brain, with the approximate location of major functions.

We do not mean to oversimplify or suggest that the prefrontal cortex is the only area of the brain related to executive skills. Recent neuroimaging evidence suggests that other areas of the brain also are involved (Pliszka, 2002). Nonetheless, the prefrontal cortex and nearby associated systems play a preeminent role in the relationship between brain structure and executive function (Bronson, 2000).

Prefrontal brain systems are among the last to fully develop, in late adolescence, and they are the final, common pathway for managing information and behavior from other brain regions. Hart and Jacobs (1993) have summarized the critical functions of the frontal lobes in the management of information and behavior:

1. The frontal lobes decide what is worth attending to and what is worth doing.
2. The frontal lobes provide continuity and coherence to behavior across time.
3. The frontal lobes modulate affective and interpersonal behaviors so that drives are satisfied within the constraints of the internal and external environments.
4. The frontal lobes monitor, evaluate, and adjust. (pp. 2, 3)

Thus, the executive skills that we have defined above are intimately tied to the frontal lobes and more broadly to frontal brain systems. This relationship can help us understand how executive skills develop over the course of childhood. It also can help us understand how executive skills can be affected by factors such as attention-deficit/hyperactivity disorder (ADHD) or brain injury.

SEQUENCE OF DEVELOPMENT

At birth we do not have executive skills that are developed or available for use. Instead, they lie dormant in the brain as future skills, in much the same way language does. Assuming there is no insult to the brain and that experience is reasonably normal, these skills will unfold over time. But as they unfold, they are influenced by the genes that we inherit from our parents as well as by the biological and social environment in which we live. If our parents did not have good organization or attention skills, chances are increased that we will have executive skill problems. If we are raised in a biologically or socially toxic environment (e.g., where lead exposure or psychological trauma takes place), there is an increased likelihood that our executive skills will suffer. However, assuming that no genetic or environmental disasters take place, executive skills will begin to develop and show themselves soon after birth in a slow progression to full adult development.

Of the theories of executive function, we favor the model proposed by Barkley (1997) in which he attempts to provide a sequence for the development of these skills beginning in infancy (Figure 1.2). Barkley's model contains five essential elements: behavioral inhibition; working memory (nonverbal); self regulation of affect/motivation/arousal; internalization of speech (verbal working memory); and reconstitution (Barkley, 1997, p.191). The cornerstone of this model is behavioral inhibition, which begins to emerge in the 5- to 12-month age range. This first executive function has three properties that allow us to delay or stop a behavior:

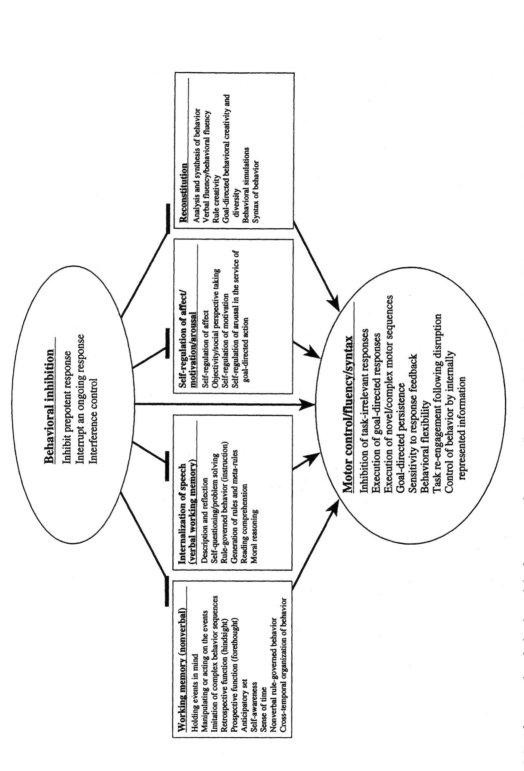

Behavioral inhibition

Inhibit prepotent response
Interrupt an ongoing response
Interference control

Working memory (nonverbal)

Holding events in mind
Manipulating or acting on the events
Imitation of complex behavior sequences
Retrospective function (hindsight)
Prospective function (forethought)
Anticipatory set
Self-awareness
Sense of time
Nonverbal rule-governed behavior
Cross-temporal organization of behavior

Internalization of speech (verbal working memory)

Description and reflection
Self-questioning/problem solving
Rule-governed behavior (instruction)
Generation of rules and meta-rules
Reading comprehension
Moral reasoning

Self-regulation of affect/ motivation/arousal

Self-regulation of affect
Objectivity/social perspective taking
Self-regulation of motivation
Self-regulation of arousal in the service of goal-directed action

Reconstitution

Analysis and synthesis of behavior
Verbal fluency/behavioral fluency
Rule creativity
Goal-directed behavioral creativity and diversity
Behavioral simulations
Syntax of behavior

Motor control/fluency/syntax

Inhibition of task-irrelevant responses
Execution of goal-directed responses
Execution of novel/complex motor sequences
Goal-directed persistence
Sensitivity to response feedback
Behavioral flexibility
Task re-engagement following disruption
Control of behavior by internally represented information

FIGURE 1.2. The complete hybrid model of executive functions (boxes) and the relationship of these four functions to the behavioral inhibition and motor control systems. From Barkley (1997, p. 191). Copyright 1997 by The Guilford Press. Reprinted by permission.

1. *The ability to delay or prevent the response leading to an immediate consequence so that some later occurring consequence may impact behavior* ("I won't make this sarcastic comment now which would annoy my teacher. I'll listen quietly so she'll respond positively to me later").
2. *The ability to stop ongoing behaviors when they prove unsuccessful* ("The comments I'm making are not getting a positive response from my teacher").
3. *The ability to manage distractions or interruptions that could interfere with the work of other executive skills* ("I need to move away from my friend because his comments are distracting me from keeping in mind what my teacher is saying").

Thus, *behavioral inhibition* helps us to think before we act and to decide when and if we will respond. It precedes the other executive functions and shields them from interference. If we didn't have inhibition, it is easy to see that our ability to use planning, goal-directed persistence, and the like would be very difficult. For the infant, inhibition is the first and most basic step in self-control because it gives the infant the power to respond or not respond to a person or event. Throughout life we use this ability to stop or delay a response as a way both to manage our own behavior and to influence the behavior of others.

While behavioral inhibition gives the infant some control over what to respond to (e.g., "I can respond or not respond to this person in front of me making the funny face"), the infant remains stuck in the present. Without some type of memory, some ability to represent real people and events in the mind, the infant can only respond to what she can see/hear/touch etc., right now, in this place right here. This sets the stage for the next executive skill in the Barkley model, *nonverbal working memory*. Development of this skill begins in the 5- to 12-month age range and involves the ability to hold information "on line" in the mind. This gives the infant the rudimentary capacity to move beyond "right now" and "right here." Nonverbal working memory becomes the foundation for the child's ability to make decisions and control behavior even though a person or an activity is not present here or now. As information and experience increase, the child develops the ability to look backward and forward ("hindsight" and "forethought"; Barkley, 1997, pp. 165–166), to mentally manipulate events, and to imitate more complex behaviors. With the expansion of her mental life, the child becomes less tied to the events and consequences of the immediate situation, of here-and-now "real life." Because of this, behavior can be brought under control of mental representations ("Last Saturday, after I finished cleaning my room, Mom took me and a friend out for pizza. I'll ask her if we can do that again after I clean my room."). Obviously the infant does not have this capacity but, in the ability to hold a picture of mother in her mind, we can see the beginnings of this control.

The third skill in Barkley's model is self-regulation of affect/motivation/arousal (Barkley, 1997, p. 211). The earliest manifestation of this skill comes in the 5-month range and becomes more evident when locomotion develops. It involves a number of subskills including regulation of emotional and motivational states, regulation of arousal, and the capacity for social perspective taking. We can begin to see how the development of this skill can give emotional and motivational value to the mental representations that the child is forming in working memory. Initially, for example, the child sees mother's face and associates this stimulus with a feeling of pleasure or comfort. With the representation of mother's face in working memory, the child can experience the pleasure in the absence of the "real" stimulus and be motivated/aroused to seek mother. Thus, the pleasurable representation triggers a drive that leads to a motor response. Behavioral inhibition may come into play when the child crosses paths with a potential distracting stimulus (e.g., a favored toy) but is able to ignore this and continue in pursuit of the original goal. As the child's representational experiences grow and acquire emotional value, and as hindsight and forethought expand across time, choices multiply and the child is freed from control by the immediate environment. Longer-term goals (from the infant's search for mother to the teenager's search for a college) become increasingly more powerful factors in setting a behavioral direction. Language is the next factor to significantly enhance this capacity.

Internalization of speech is the next of the executive skills to develop, according to Barkley (1997, p. 174). Acquisition of language provides the child with a powerful tool for control of the environment. People, objects, and actions and the images of these that the child has formed in nonverbal working memory can now be represented with words. More importantly, these words provide the child with a means for exercising some control over the world. It is no longer necessary for the child to walk to mother or point to what he wants. Instead he can use his words to accomplish what previously took physical actions. Language also becomes an increasingly powerful means for adults (and other children) to regulate the child's behavior. What begins as management of behavior by the language of other people gradually shifts in part to self-management. Initially, the child accomplishes this by adopting the adult words and publicly saying them to himself. According to Barkley, this self-speech is evident in the 3- to 5-year-old and becomes increasingly more private or covert until it is largely internalized by 9 to 12 years. This skill involves much more than basic self-control. Over time, internalization of speech facilitates the development of rules, problem-solving strategies, self-monitoring, self-instruction, and metacognition.

The final element to develop in the Barkley model is reconstitution, defined as the "analysis and synthesis of behavior" (1997, p. 185). This executive skill enables the individual to divide more complex behavioral sequences into component units (analysis) and recombine them in novel ways (synthesis) to solve new problems or reach new goals. Hence, reconstitution represents cognitive and behavioral flexibility, fluency, and creativity. Barkley sees this skill as representing the capacity for covert rehearsal or simulation before making a decision on how best to proceed. Thus, it is an opportunity for the child to find a good fit between a problem or goal and a behavioral strategy. This obviously is a more sophisticated and later developing skill that, based on research about children's planning ability, emerges in its early stages at about 6 years.

These skills, then, are critical if children are to develop complex independent living and problem-solving abilities. Although executive skills begin to emerge in early infancy, they reach a reasonable level of development only by mid-to-late adolescence. It is at this point that relevant adults (parents, teachers, employers) begin to feel more confidence in the self-regulatory ability of the teenager. This increased confidence is reflected in the options and opportunities that we make available to teens, such as a driver's license, less restricted work hours, course selection, and credit cards. Prior to this development, adults help compensate for incomplete development by "lending" their frontal lobes or executive skills to the child.

This happens in one of two ways. The first is direct, coming in the form of directives, limits, and rules. For example, in the toddler who has little impulse control, moving toward potential danger typically leads to a sharp "No!" Or for the young child who is unable to make and follow a plan, we, the adults, construct the plan and then prompt or cue each step, not completing the task for the child but ensuring that with help he or she is successful. In effect, we are a surrogate frontal lobe that operates for the child as a set of supplementary executive skills. However, we are not there indefinitely to provide these skills to children. Rather, we are there to prompt and to teach them, and then to step back as their own executive skills unfold. The second method involves structuring the environment in a way that compensates for underdeveloped skills. For example, with toddlers we use gates to prohibit entry or escape. We order the environment and label it with pictures or words to help organization. For adolescents we gate off, as best we can, access to alcohol, drugs, and weapons. And we attempt to hold them in a controlled environment—school—where their options only gradually expand. This model is not universal, but it certainly prevails in Western cultures (and gradually emerges in developing countries).

DEVELOPMENTAL TASKS REQUIRING EXECUTIVE SKILLS

Let's move from theory to a concrete description of the kinds of tasks children and teenagers perform that require executive skills. Table 1.1 lists specific tasks or behaviors adults commonly expect children to be able to perform in different age ranges. In reviewing this table, the reader should keep in mind that there are developmental variations between children such that at any given age some children can perform tasks at an independent level while other children will require cuing, supervision, or even assistance to perform the same tasks. This table should be considered as approximate rather than explicit guidelines for behavioral expectations at any age level.

Determining the level of a child's executive skills in relation to these developmental tasks can help us to understand the "goodness of fit" between the child and his or her world. This assessment in turn can help us to judge the adjustments that may be needed in the degree of "frontal lobe" support provided by adults, whether modifications in adult expectations are called for, and whether environmental supports should be added or withdrawn. Such an assessment also sets the stage for determining the next set of skills to be taught as well as how these executive skills can be shaped to promote both success and independence.

TABLE 1.1. Developmental Tasks Requiring Executive Skills

Age range	Developmental task
Preschool	Run simple errands (e.g., "Get your shoes from the bedroom").
	Tidy bedroom or playroom with assistance.
	Perform simple chores and self-help tasks with reminders (e.g., clear dishes from table, brush teeth, get dressed).
	Inhibit behaviors: don't touch a hot stove; don't run into the street; don't grab a toy from another child; don't hit, bite, push, etc.
Kindergarten–grade 2	Run errands (two to three step directions).
	Tidy bedroom or playroom.
	Perform simple chores, self-help tasks; may need reminders (e.g., make bed).
	Bring papers to and from school.
	Complete homework assignments (20-minute maximum).
	Decide how to spend money (allowance).
	Inhibit behaviors: follow safety rules, don't swear, raise hand before speaking in class, keep hands to self.
Grades 3–5	Run errands (may involve time delay or greater distance, such as going to a nearby store or remembering to do something after school).
	Tidy bedroom or playroom (may include vacuuming, dusting, etc.).
	Perform chores that take 15–30 minutes (e.g., clean up after dinner, rake leaves).
	Bring books, papers, assignments to and from school.
	Keep track of belongings when away from home.
	Complete homework assignments (1 hour maximum).
	Plan simple school project such as book reports (select book, read book, write report).
	Keep track of changing daily schedule (i.e., different activities after school).
	Save money for desired objects, plan how to earn money.
	Inhibit/self-regulate: behave when teacher is out of the classroom; refrain from rude comments, temper tantrums, bad manners.
Grades 6–8	Help out with chores around the home, including both daily responsibilities and occasional tasks (e.g., emptying dishwasher, raking leaves, shoveling snow); tasks may take 60–90 minutes to complete.
	Baby-sit younger siblings or for pay.
	Use system for organizing schoolwork, including assignment book, notebooks, etc.
	Follow complex school schedule involving changing teachers and changing schedules.
	Plan and carry out long-term projects, including tasks to be accomplished and reasonable timeline to follow; may require planning multiple large projects simultaneously.
	Plan time, including after school activities, homework, family responsibilities; estimate how long it takes to complete individual tasks and adjust schedule to fit.
	Inhibit rule breaking in the absence of visible authority.

(continued)

TABLE 1.1. (*continued*)

Age range	Developmental task
High school	Manage schoolwork effectively on a day-to-day basis, including completing and handing in assignments on time, studying for tests, creating and following timelines for long-term projects, and making adjustments in effort and quality of work in response to feedback from teachers and others (e.g., grades on tests, papers).
	Establish and refine a long-term goal and make plans for meeting that goal. If the goal beyond high school is college, the youngster selects appropriate courses and maintains grade point average (GPA) to ensure acceptance into college. The youngster also participates in extracurricular activities, signs up for and takes Scholastic Aptitude Tests (SATs) or American College Tests (ACTs) at the appropriate time and carries out the college application process. If the youngster does not plan to go to college, he or she pursues vocational courses and, if applicable, employment outside of school to ensure the training and experience necessary to obtain employment after graduation.
	Make good use of leisure time, including obtaining employment or pursuing recreational activities during the summer.
	Inhibit reckless and dangerous behaviors (e.g., use of illegal substances, sexual acting out, shoplifting, or vandalism).

2

Assessing Executive Skills

For those who are accustomed to using standardized measures to assess processing disorders or learning disabilities, the assessment of executive functions presents a somewhat different challenge. It is possible to assess language-based learning disorders, nonverbal learning disabilities, and dyslexia using instruments such as tests of intelligence, achievement, language, memory, and phonological processing—tests that are normed on a typical population of students—with a diagnosis deriving from a distinct cognitive profile or a discrepancy between ability and specific academic achievement measures.

Accurate assessment of executive skills is essential for effective intervention for two primary reasons. First, as noted, executive skills are intimately related to the frontal regions of the brain and these frontal brain regions represent a final common pathway for much of human behavior. Because of this, a variety of different factors may affect executive skills. For example, depression, anxiety, fatigue, situational stress, or an attention disorder, among others, can adversely impact executive skills. Alternatively, a child may have inherent weaknesses in one or more executive skills, unrelated to other factors. Understanding the reason for the weakness is critical for determining the most effective intervention, especially since interventions will differ widely depending on the source of the weakness. An antidepressant medication is unlikely to resolve an inherent weakness in organization. Conversely, templates for organization are unlikely to resolve a problem whose source is low energy resulting from sadness.

The second key reason for accurate assessment is the need to understand the pattern of strengths and weaknesses in a child's executive skills. Without such information, attempts to intervene are nonspecific and hence likely to miss the mark. For example, in the absence of an executive skills assessment, a child may well be mismatched with her environment and taught skills she does not need, while critical skills are neglected. At best, such an approach is inefficient. At worst, it is a source of frustration and anger for the child, parents, and teachers. Thus accurate assessment of executive skills is key to efficient. effective strategies for intervention.

Attempting to assess executive skills in the context of a formal evaluation is difficult, however, because so many of the factors that demand the use of executive skills on the part of the student are removed from the equation. Just some examples of why this is the case follow:

1. Two critical executive skills are initiation and sustained attention. In standardized testing situations, the examiner cues the student to start and presents tasks that are necessarily brief in nature, thereby reducing the demand for sustained attention.

2. Standardized testing situations require the presence of an adult performing a monitoring function. With the tester performing this role, the student does not have to monitor his or her own performance to the same extent, a critical executive skill.

3. In the context of a highly structured, if not ritualized, set of tasks, the need for planning and organization on the part of the student is reduced, if not in many cases eliminated.

4. Executive skills are most in demand in the face of complex, open-ended tasks requiring problem solving and creative or unique solutions. Standardized tests are designed to be easily scored with a catalog of right and wrong answers that are straightforward and invariant, again minimizing demands on executive skills.

5. The most complex cognitive task within any psychologist's repertoire is less complex than real-world demands on executive skills, and there is no way of determining with any certainty how well these tests map on to the real world. Thus, in the parlance of neuropsychologists, *absence of evidence is not evidence of absence*. In other words, a child's strong performance on a clinic measure of executive function (say, the Tower test described below) does not necessarily mean that that same child applies good planning ability in the context of daily performance at home or at school.

Best practice in the assessment of executive function must therefore extend beyond the use of formal standardized measures. While such measures may have a place in the evaluation process, assessing executive skills, we believe, can benefit from several additional sources of information, both informal and standardized. These include: (1) a detailed case history with interview questions designed to elicit the presence or absence of executive skills in everyday activities, (2) classroom observations, (3) work samples, and (4) standardized behavior rating scales. These elements will be discussed below.

INFORMAL ASSESSMENT MEASURES

Case History/Interview

A critical piece of the process when assessing a youngster's executive functioning is to gather information from those who know the child best, usually parents and teachers. When we interview parents, we ask questions about how the child manages homework and other chores and responsibilities at home. For instance:

Can he plan tasks on his own?

Does she need reminders to get started on homework?

Does he need encouragement to keep working until the job is done?

Does she need constant supervision to ensure task completion?

How does he handle morning or bedtime routines—can he follow them independently or does he need cues and reminders?

We ask how organized the child is:

Does she keep her bedroom or study area neat?

Does he know where to find belongings?

Does she keep notebooks and backpacks organized?

And we ask questions about the child's ability to control her behavior—with friends, with siblings, with parents, when frustrated, when stressed, when disappointed. All of these questions tell us something about the youngster's ability to plan and organize, initiate tasks, and sustain attention, as well as her ability to regulate her behavior when confronted with obstacles.

Teachers can provide us similar information. When we interview teachers, we ask them how well the student in question is able to work independently, how well he organizes and keeps track of materials and possessions in school, and how well he plans and executes activities. And, again, we ask about the student's ability to manage behavior when stressed and his ability to control impulses.

With older students (and some more insightful younger ones), we ask them similar questions. We ask about common homework problems, their ability to plan for long-term projects, how they study for tests, and what organizational strategies they use to keep track of things. We also ask about leisure time activities: Do they use their time well, or do they tend to spend too much time engaged in certain activities—hanging out with friends, instant messaging, playing computer and video games? We may also ask them how they manage negative emotions: Do siblings, parents, or other kids get on their nerves? What do they do when an assignment frustrates them? And so on.

The objective is to complete a mini-functional assessment to determine (1) specific behaviors that demonstrate strong/weak executive skills, (2) circumstances (people, places, times) under which the problems are most/least likely to occur, (3) previous successful/unsuccessful interventions, and (4) capacity/receptivity of the people and/or environment to change. Obviously not all questions may be answered during the interview, but in the same sense that the assessment process leads to generation and clarification of hypotheses about skills, it also leads to generation and clarification of possible interventions. For example, knowing that a parent is organizationally challenged or that a teacher already feels overwhelmed by demands on her or his time can lead to different decisions about intervention.

The Appendix contains structured interview forms that can be used with parents, teachers, and students to assess executive skills. Because the questionnaires are intended to be used in the course of interviews, the questions on all three questionnaires are organized around common problem areas that students have rather than organized around specific executive skill deficits. However, to facilitate identifying specific executive skill deficits, each question is coded with the executive skill it is believed to tap. These three sources provide us with rich clinical data about how parents, teachers, and youngsters themselves view executive functioning. From these data alone, we can begin to formulate some environmental modifications and behavioral interventions, but we find it helpful to add normative data to this mix as well.

Classroom Observations

Classroom observation by the examiner can play a key role in assessment and intervention since it provides the opportunity to see executive skills in their most important context— the daily demands of school. It is within the setting of the classroom environment or classroom demands (e.g., homework) that executive skills problems often are first noted and the success of any intervention will be judged by an observed change in behavior. Hence, a classroom observation sets the stage for a clear definition of the executive skill as a specific behavior, points to the direction for intervention, and provides the gold standard for evaluating effectiveness (i.e., did the behavior change?). In conducting the observation, the setting events, antecedents, and responses to the behavior may all be visible to the observer, along with the impact of potential interventions (Table 2.1).

A second alternative is to have the teacher, aide, or another specialist (e.g., school psychologist, counselor, or occupational therapist) collect some of the data. For this to be feasible, data collection methods need to fit easily within the schedule of the classroom and the person observing, particularly if it is the teacher. Fortunately, a number of executive skills involve production (homework, classwork, projects), so that work samples (see below for more details) or the absence of them are a readily available "permanent product measure" that can be used to assess behavior. For other executive skill weaknesses, the type of behavior will determine the observation method. For example, the length of time needed to begin a task, the percentage of time on task, and the numbers of times speaking out will serve as reliable measures of task initiation, sustained attention, and response inhibition, respectively.

As noted above, observed behavior or its product in natural, everyday settings ultimately will constitute the best measure of an executive skill. A change in the behavior will constitute the best measure of an effective intervention. Prior to intervention, the person seeking the change (parent, teacher, student) must come to an agreement with the person planning the intervention about what outcome behavior will need to be observed to define success.

Work Samples

Work samples such as tests, writing assignments, and agenda pages can help assess skills such as error monitoring, planning, and organization and yield ideas for interventions such as cue questions and templates. Work samples might also include looking at the child's backpack or desk to get a better sense of the child's ability to organize his or her personal space.

TABLE 2.1. Tips for Doing Classroom Observations

- Complete interviews and rating scales prior to scheduling the classroom observation. This gives the evaluator a good idea about the problem areas and in what classroom situations they are likely to be observed.

- Identify with the classroom teacher what his or her primary concerns are and identify the times or classroom activities in which the behaviors of concern are most likely to be observed. Let the teacher know whether he or she should intervene as is typically done (e.g., redirecting the child to get back to work) or if the teacher should not intervene so that the observer can get an idea of how the child behaves when left "on his own."

- Sit behind the target child or off to the side, in a location where the child cannot make easy eye contact with the observer.

- Collect both objective data (e.g., percentage of time on task) as well as a running record of the child's behavior throughout the observation.

- In addition to observing the child, observe the physical environment to determine if there are factors about the classroom space that might be contributing to the problem or could be changed to reduce the problem. Watch the teacher to see how he or she cues the child or manages the classroom routines. This information could prove valuable when planning interventions.

- It is useful to compare the target child to other children in the class. This can be done either by asking the teacher to point out a "typical" child to be observed at the same time the target child is observed or by watching the entire class in a systematic way. For example, if collecting "time on task" data using an interval recording procedure, then alternate intervals should be directed toward another child in the class, rotating through the entire class during the observation period.

- Arrange, if time permits, to come back and observe on another day. Several short observations spread over several days may be more useful than one long observation on a single day.

- Be sure to check back with the teacher after the observation to determine whether the behavior observed was typical or atypical of the child.

- Observe the child in settings other than the classroom. This is particularly important if the child's problems relate to poor impulse control or regulation of affect, since these behaviors are likely to be more evident in less structured situations such as in the hallways, in the cafeteria, or out at recess.

BEHAVIOR CHECKLISTS

Several behavior rating scales provide information regarding executive skills in children and adolescents. A sample of these are discussed below.

Behavior Rating Inventory of Executive Functions

Available from Psychological Assessment Resources, the Behavior Rating Inventory of Executive Functions (BRIEF; Gioia, Isquith, Guy, & Kenworthy, 2000) was normed on children ages 5–18 and includes both parent and teacher versions. It is an 86-item inventory in which the parent or teacher is asked to determine on a 3-point scale how often the child performs the problem behavior (never, sometimes, always). The scale yields a global measure of executive functioning as well as two indexes, Behavioral Regulation and Metacognition, and eight scales assessing individual executive skills. The Behavioral Regulation Index includes three subscales, Inhibit, Shift, and Emotional Control, while the Metacognition Index includes five scales: Initiate, Working Memory, Plan/Organize, Organization of Materials, and Monitor.

Brown ADD Scales—Adolescent Version

Available from the Psychological Corporation, this rating scale (Brown, 1996) is intended for use as a component of a structured interview designed to assess attention-deficit disorders (ADDs). There are a total of 40 items which fall into five clusters: Activation, Attention, Effort, Affect, and Memory. The test is normed on high school students, with the total score falling into one of three ranges: ADD possible but not likely, ADD probable but not certain, and ADD highly probable. The individual clusters quite readily translate into broader executive skills (e.g., self-regulation of affect, working memory, initiation, sustained attention, and goal-directed persistence).

Comprehensive Behavior Rating Scale for Children

Also available from the Psychological Corporation, the Comprehensive Behavior Rating Scale for Children (CBRSC; Neeper, Lahey, & Frick, 1990) is normed on children ages 6–14 and yields eight separate scale scores. Several of the scales, particularly Inattention/Disorganization and Motoric Hyperactivity include items that tap a number of executive skills including sustained attention, working memory, organization, and inhibition. Here are some examples of specific items: *Can do only one thing at a time. Forgets sequences of instructions. Has difficulty with tasks that require sustained attention. Responds to questions before thinking through answers. Becomes disorganized when changing from one task to another. Seems scatterbrained or confused. Is unable to organize and focus on a specific task.*

Child Behavior Checklist—Teacher Report Form

These rating scales were developed by Thomas M. Achenbach (1991b) and his colleagues and are designed as a broad measures of social-emotional functioning. Specific items tap executive skills, particularly those included on the Attention Problems scale. In addition, however, these measures are useful for the open-ended questions included on the form. For instance, the Teacher Report Form asks the teacher to indicate both the "best things about this pupil," and "what concerns you most about this pupil?" Answers to these questions can provide insight into the teacher's perceptions of a child's executive skills depending on the nature of the responses.

FORMAL ASSESSMENT MEASURES

Formal assessment serves a number of functions. It provides the context for examining other variables such as cognitive abilities, emotional status, and academic skills that may well impact and be impacted by executive skills. In complex cases (see Chapter 7) formal assessment can play a key role in intervention planning and prioritization, in some cases relegating executive skill problems to the "back burner" until more significant factors are addressed. Formal assessment also can provide a minilaboratory, allowing the evaluator to see how a skill weakness manifests itself and what impact, if any, interventions such as cuing, rehearsal, or external structure may have on the child's behavior.

Only a few tests have been designed specifically to assess the broad array of executive skills as we have defined them here. Below is a list of tests and subtests which can be used to assess individual executive skills, including a description of the task and the skills it is designed to assess.

NEPSY

The NEPSY (Korkman, Kirk, & Kemp, 1998) is an individually administered battery that includes a number of subtests designed to assess executive skills in children, including planning, cognitive flexibility, impulsivity, vigilance, auditory selective attention, monitoring, self-regulation, and problem solving.

Porteus Mazes

This maze tracing task (Porteus, 1959), according to its developer, was designed to investigate "the process of choosing, trying, and rejecting or adopting a very complex maze" (p. 7). To be successful, the person must trace the maze and not enter any blind alley or go through any solid wall.

Matching Familiar Figures Test

This visual matching task (Kagan, 1966) involves rapidly comparing a stimulus picture with one of six very similar response figures, only one of which is a correct match. Latency to first response and errors are measured, and the test is designed to assess reflectivity/impulsivity.

Trailmaking Tests

These visual–motor tasks (Reitan & Wolfson, 1985) require rapid graphomotor sequencing of numbers and then alternating number–letter patterns on a page. The tests involve visual scanning and attention, motor speed, and cognitive flexibility or the ability to establish and change mental set.

Wisconsin Card Sorting Test

The Wisconsin Card Sorting Test (Heaton, 1981) is a conceptual sorting task that requires the individual to sort cards with four different types and numbers of symbols on them according to one of four stimulus cards. These stimulus cards represent the sorting categories (e.g., color, shape, or number). The test is designed to evaluate the individual's ability to establish and shift mental set.

Mesulam Tests of Directed Attention

This is a pencil-and-paper cancellation test (Mesulam, 1985) in which the student is asked to locate target letters in ordered and random letter arrays. Although this is a brief task, it is somewhat tedious. To do well requires sustained attention, planning skills to devise a search strategy, and self-monitoring to evaluate performance and determine when the task is finished.

Conners Continuous Performance Test—II

This is a computerized attention task (Conners, 2000) in which the student watches letters flash on the computer screen and is instructed to press the space bar or the mouse button for every letter except a specific target letter (X). The task requires sustained attention and the ability to inhibit a motor response.

Delis–Kaplan Executive Function Scale

This is an individually administered battery of nine tests (Delis, Kaplan, & Kramer, 2000) designed to assess a range of different executive skills in children and adults. The tests assess executive functions including planning, cognitive flexibility, impulsivity, and problem solving.

Cognitive Assessment System

This individually administered cognitive test (Naglieri & Das, 1997) uses six subtests to determine performance on two scales, Planning and Attention, which involve executive functions. The Planning subtests require strategy use for efficient problem solution. The Attention subtests demand sustained concentration for target detection and avoidance of distractions.

BEHAVIORAL OBSERVATIONS WITH FORMAL ASSESSMENT MEASURES

While test scores can provide insight into a child's level of executive functioning, the richest source of information available through formal assessment may be the child's behavior during the evaluation process. What follows is a brief discussion of how an examiner may gain information about executive functioning while observing a student's response to specific tasks or to testing in general.

Self-Regulation of Affect

Formal tests are often frustrating for students because they are designed to become more difficult as the task goes along. How children respond to the challenge presented by progressively more difficult tasks can offer insight into their ability to regulate their emotions. The child who gives up quickly, pushes test materials away, or refuses to continue is likely a child who has difficulty managing emotions in the face of stress.

Metacognition

Metacognitive skills are most apparent in a test situation in those children who talk their way through difficult tasks. This self-talk provides for the examiner a window to the student's capacity to use thought to solve problems and respond to challenge. Some students will engage in self-instruction ("first I do this, then I do this," etc.), others will self-monitor ("no, that's not right, I have to fix that"), while yet others will self-evaluate ("you dummy, you did it wrong!"). With students who don't talk aloud, the examiner may want to ask them what they did to solve a particularly difficult problem.

Goal-Directed Persistence

Because formal tests necessarily present the student with comparatively brief tasks, goal-directed persistence can only be assessed in the context of short time periods and simple tasks. Youngsters who are determined to solve difficult puzzles will provide some insight into their capacity to persist in the face of obstacles, but it is not wise to generalize too much from this kind of testing situation when assessing a student's capacity to persist over time to achieve a goal.

Flexibility

Some tasks lend themselves to the assessment of flexibility. Tasks requiring puzzle completion, for instance, often involve "false starts" or the need for a change in strategy. The Comprehension subtest of the Wechsler Intelligence Scale for Children—Third Edition (WISC-III; Wechsler, 1991) has a number of items that require the student to provide more than one answer to a question (e.g., "Tell me some reasons why dogs make good pets"). Many tests include early items where, if the student makes a mistake, the examiner corrects the mistake. Observing his or her response to that correction can provide the examiner with a sense of the student's flexibility in the face of corrective feedback.

Sustained Attention

A good way to assess this capacity is to include a variety of tasks, some more interesting than others, within an evaluation. The Kaufman Assessment Battery for Children, for instance, does this well with quite young children since some of the tasks are more appealing than others and some require close attention to comparatively uninteresting information.

Working Memory

Tasks that require working memory include those that involve mental arithmetic and those that require the manipulation of information as well as recall, such as the digits backward condition of the WISC-III Digit Span subtest. If the child asks to have arithmetic questions repeated, this suggests the possibility of weak working memory.

Response Inhibition

Problems with this executive skill are apparent in a number of ways. Youngsters may blurt out answers before the question is completed, announce that they are "done" on puzzle tasks and then discover that they made a mistake, reach for materials before the examiner has finished laying them out, or, in the case of the Object Assembly subtest of the WISC-III, peek over the screen as the examiner sets out the puzzle pieces.

Planning/Prioritization

This executive skill does not lend itself to assessment through formal measures. It may be possible to obtain some insights about a person's planning capacity through watching how she performs on mazes (e.g., Porteus Mazes or the Mazes subtest of the WISC-III), how she completes tasks such as the Tower subtest of the NEPSY, or how she draws the Rey–Osterrieth Complex Figure, but it would be dangerous to make inferences about real-life planning skills from any of these subtests.

Time Management

We do not know of tests or subtests that assess this capacity well.

Organization

The same tasks assessing planning (described above) have an organization component to them. We repeat the cautions associated with interpreting results.

Task Initiation

Because the examiner acts as a cue for task initiation in any formal testing situation, this is not well assessed in this manner.

To reiterate what we have stated in this chapter: The primary value in formal assessment of executive skills is as a medium for the clinical observation of those skills. Tests provide the examiner with a structured set of skill demands for the child. Careful behavioral observation of the child as she attempts to meet those demands can provide valuable information about executive skills (is there evidence of planning, organization, ability to sustain attention, impulse control, etc.?). Test scores, in and of themselves, do not provide this information, and to expect therefore that formal test data will yield definitive answers regarding executive skill deficits is a mistake. Scores alone, whether above or below average, do not reliably determine the presence or absence of executive skills. We are not suggesting that test scores be ignored or that they have no value. Rather, we believe that observation of the process by the evaluator informs and validates formal assessment data. Finally, we have noted that the presence of the evaluator and the structure of the situation diminish the executive skill demands on the child. Hence, the information gathered in formal assessment must be judged against the child's performance in everyday situations if the evaluation is to have validity.

CASE EXAMPLE

To illustrate the assessment process, we now present a brief case example in which a variety of assessment techniques were incorporated. The assessment procedure is described along with the information obtained from that procedure.

Parent Interview/Developmental History Forms

Scott is a 10-year-old child living with his parents and older brother and attending a small private school. Birth history was unremarkable and developmental milestones were within normal limits. There is no significant family or medical history. Scott has attended the same school since preschool, and according to parent reports, teachers noted a tendency to wander around the classroom and to have difficulty initiating activities as early as preschool. In kindergarten, problems with activity level, concentration, and distractibility were all reported. Parents initiated an evaluation because teachers were reporting continuing problems with task initiation and work completion, as well as concerns about motor restlessness and impulsivity.

At home, Scott's parents describe him as an active child who prefers to be outdoors or on the go. He has difficulty sitting through meals and requires frequent reminders to complete chores and follow morning routines. He is able to engage in both reading and television viewing for long periods of time with no apparent attention problems. Homework completion, however, is problematic both due to difficulty getting started on homework and seeing it through to completion. Scott has friends outside of school with whom he plays regularly. However, his parents note that he has some difficulty interpreting social cues and he seems to have difficulty "fitting into a group." He tends to be literal, overly concrete, and lacks flexibility.

Teacher Interview

In an interview the evaluator conducted with Scott's teachers, they describe him as an active child who has an almost constant need to be "moving or touching someone." Hence, boundary issues with peers arise frequently and require teacher attention and mediation.

His impulsivity can extend to his work, resulting in messy papers, broken pens/pencils, and cluttered spaces. Other than fiction reading, he has difficulty with initiation and completion of work, especially if it involves written output. At the same time, they see him as a boy who is curious about almost any subject and eager to learn. His teachers feel that if he could better manage his impulsivity and task focus, there would be significant improvements in peer relationships and academics.

Behavior Rating Scales

Scott's parents completed the Child Behavior Checklist (Achenbach, 1991a), placing Scott in the clinical range on the scale as a whole and on the Social Problems and the Attention Problems subscales. They also completed that ADHD Rating Scale, Home Version (DuPaul, Power, Anastopoulos, & Reid, 1998) and placed Scott in the clinical range (i.e., above the 93rd percentile) on both the Inattention and Hyperactive subscales. His teachers placed him in the clinical range on the Externalizing Problems of the Child Behavior Checklist—Teacher Report Form (Achenbach, 1991b) and in the borderline clinical range on the scale as a whole and on the Hyperactivity/Impulsivity subscale. The placed him below the clinical range on the ADHD Rating Scale, School Version (DuPaul et al., 1998). However, on the Comprehensive Behavior Rating Scale for Children (Neeper et al., 1990), teachers placed him in the clinical range on the Motoric Hyperactivity and the Oppositional/Conduct Disorders subscales.

Parents and teachers also completed the Behavior Rating Inventory of Executive Function (Gioia et al., 2000). His parents placed him in the clinical range on the total scale, on the Metacognitive Index, and on five of eight subscales (Shift, Initiate, Working Memory, Plan/Organize, Monitor). His teachers placed him in the clinical range on the scale as a whole, on both the Behavior Regulation Index and the Metacognitive Index and all eight subscales (Inhibit, Emotional Control, and Organization of Materials, in addition to those the parents reported).

Taken as a whole, parents and teachers both reported significant executive skill weaknesses. Parents also reported significant attention problems and social problems, but these dimensions were rated as less problematic by teachers. Teachers, however, reported higher levels of acting out or externalizing behaviors, perhaps associated with impulsivity and overactivity.

Behavioral Observations

Scott was observed in his classroom during two periods, one involving independent math work and the other a teacher-led discussion with students sitting in a circle. Percentage of time on task was assessed during the 15-minute independent period. Scott was compared to a male peer judged by the teacher to have average attention. Scott was on task 35% of the time in comparison to 75% for the other boy. In addition to moving around frequently, Scott intermittently made random, low-level sounds. During the teacher-led activity, frequency of physical contact with nearby peers (touching, bumping, laying against them) was measured using an interval recording technique. Scott was in physical contact with other students during 55% of the intervals in comparison to 10% for a matched peer.

During the evaluation session, Scott presented as initially quiet and serious, but he became more talkative as the session went along. He tended to respond quickly to questions, his initial answers often being both impulsive and incorrect. Careless mistakes due to inattention were observed, particularly on visual tasks, and he failed to check his work for accuracy.

Formal Assessment Results

Both as a device for facilitating behavioral observations and because his parents were interested in obtaining information about Scott's learning style, cognitive, memory, and attention tasks were administered. Scott placed in the above-average range on the WISC-III (Wechsler, 1991), with verbal skills falling in the superior range and nonverbal performance skills falling in the average to above-average range. Long-term memory for verbal information was particularly strong. On visual tasks, inattention to detail affected performance on some tasks, particularly those where there was no easy way to check his work for accuracy (e.g., Picture Completion, Picture Arrangement).

Scott's performance on the subtests comprising the Memory Screening Index of the Wide Range Assessment of Memory and Learning (Sheslow & Adams, 1990) fell in the above-average to well-above-average range for the most part, but he was weaker on the Digit Span subtest of the WISC-III, considered to be a measure of working memory. On this measure, he was inconsistent in his recall of numbers in both forward and backward sequences, scoring at the low end of the average range.

Scott was administered two attention tasks. On the Mesulam Tests of Directed Attention (Mesulam, 1985), a letter cancellation task, he was asked to locate target letters in ordered and random letter arrays. Although he only missed 4 of 60 targets on the ordered array, he missed 21 of 60 targets on the random array. He spent an equal amount of time on each array, but whereas he was able to employ a systematic search strategy on the ordered array (i.e., going row by row), the random array did not lend itself to this kind of strategy. In the absence of such a search strategy, it appeared that Scott did not know how to evaluate when he was done with the task; thus he missed significantly more target letters. On a computerized attention task, Conners' Continuous Performance Test (Conners, 2000), Scott's response speed was atypically fast, suggestive of impulsivity, but he was able to sustain attention to the 15-minute task without apparent difficulty.

Conclusions

Test results indicate a bright youngster with exceptional verbal skills. The cognitive profile of significantly stronger verbal than nonverbal/visual skills suggests he may have some characteristics associated with a nonverbal learning disability, such as the cognitive rigidity his parents describe as well as difficulty reading social cues. Both verbal and visual memory skills are strong, but working memory is more problematic. Some attention problems were seen on clinic tasks. Both parents and teachers report significant problems with impulsivity and activity level, while parents also report significant problems with inattention, including distractibility, daydreaming, and difficulty concentrating. The greatest impediments to social–emotional adjustment and to academic performance at the present time appear to be related to weak executive skills, including problems with behavioral regulation (response inhibition, flexibility) as well as problems with task initiation, working memory, sustained attention, planning, and organization.

Recommendations

Scott has a number of executive skill weaknesses that warrant interventions. Priorities need to be set targeting those deficit areas that are having the biggest negative impact at the present time. Since both his parents and his teachers are primarily concerned with Scott's behavior and performance at school, designing interventions for this setting is most appropriate. Targeting impulsivity and work completion would address the most pressing needs. Strategies should include environmental modifications, a behavior plan built around an incentive system, and teaching specific skills to improve sustained attention and task completion. An intervention to address homework issues would also be warranted. These will be described in more detail in the next chapter.

3

Linking Assessment to Intervention

The goal of assessment is intervention. To meet this goal, the assessment process is designed to gather behavioral information relevant to intervention. It is not enough, however, to be able to describe the behaviors of concern in order to design an effective intervention. We must also have some understanding of why the behavior occurs. For example, a student might have difficulty completing independent classwork because he is distracted by a peer talking or because he doesn't know how to do the task (or both). Thus, throughout the assessment process we employ a hypothesis-testing approach. At each step, as information is gathered we formulate hypotheses about the environment and the child's skills that can help explain the behavior observed. By soliciting information from others and by observing the child in the natural environment and in the test environment, we refine our hypotheses and try to confirm or refute them.

This same hypothesis-testing approach can simultaneously lead to potential intervention strategies. For example, in the above example if the teacher has observed increased work completion when she is close by or when peers are not talking, the attention/distractibility hypothesis gains credibility. This information then also sets the direction for intervention. If, on the other hand, the "why" of this student's behavior is not clear, as part of our hypothesis testing we might ask the teacher to stand close by or relocate him. The outcome will help to clarify the "why" issue and the intervention strategy.

Once we have gathered our data and generated our hypotheses, the next stage in the assessment–intervention link is translation of these data into a format and plan for intervention. We have developed a process to help organize and synthesize our assessment information for the purpose of designing interventions targeted to those areas of greatest need, as defined by parents, teachers, or both. This process includes the following steps (also summarized in Table 3.1):

TABLE 3.1. Steps in Executive Skill Intervention Planning

Step 1. Collect assessment information from a variety of sources.
- Interviews
- Behavior checklists
- Classroom observations
- Work samples
- Formal assessment procedures

Step 2. Review data; list specific problem behaviors and connect them to the most appropriate executive skill domain.

Step 3. Select one executive skill domain for initial intervention and identify a specific behavioral goal (e.g., by soliciting from parents or teachers one or two behaviors, which if increased or decreased would lead to better performance for the student).

Step 4. Design the intervention, incorporating one or more of the following elements:
- Environmental supports or modifications that will be put in place to help support the development of the skill.
- The specific skills the child will be taught and the procedure used to teach them.
- What incentives will be used to help motivate the child to use or practice the skills.

Step 5. Evaluate intervention effectiveness by looking at each intervention component and answering the following questions:
- Was the component put in place?
- Was it effective?
- Does it need to be continued?
- What is the plan for fading this component?

---

1. Collect assessment information from a variety of sources, including interviews, behavior checklists, classroom observations, work samples, and formal assessment procedures.

2. Consider each executive skill in turn and identify areas of need in specific, behavioral terms. If you are not sure under which executive skill a particular behavior should be coded, include it under those that seem most relevant.

3. Determine which executive skill will be targeted for intervention first, and identify a specific behavioral goal. The following question, posed to parents or teacher may be helpful in identifying which behaviors are a priority for intervention: What are one or two behaviors, which, if they increased or decreased, would lead to say (student's name) is definitely performing better?" Identifying these behaviors should then lead to the development of a behavioral objective. This step will drive the remainder of the process including outcome evaluation criteria. According to Alberto and Troutman (1999, p. 66), there are four components to a behavioral objective. The objective should (a) *identify the learner* ("Scott will . . . "), (b) *identify the target behavior* ("complete his daily assigned homework . . . "), (c) *identify the conditions under which the behavior is to be displayed* ("between 4 and 7 P.M. with no more than two adult verbal prompts . . . "), and (d) *identify criteria for acceptable performance* ("for 90% of the assignments given during a marking period"). Once the behavioral objective is developed, a data sheet can be prepared that allows track-

ing of the behavior by the adult and the student. This data sheet can serve both as an incentive and as a way to evaluate the success of the intervention.

4. Design the intervention. Three critical elements must be considered in planning the intervention: (a) the environmental supports or modifications that will be put in place to help support development of the skill, (b) the specific skills the child will be taught and the procedure used to teach them, and (c) what incentives will be used to help motivate the child to use or practice the skills. These elements are all described in detail in Chapter 4.

5. Evaluate intervention effectiveness. This is done subsequent to putting in place the intervention. The first step in evaluating the intervention is to review the behavioral objective and assess whether the objective was achieved. Whether the objective was achieved or not, the next step is to evaluate the individual components of the intervention to determine whether they were implemented effectively. Plans for continuing, changing, or fading intervention components are made, depending on the effectiveness of the intervention. This analysis might also lead to the conclusion that the behavioral objective was unrealistic. If this is the case, a new objective should be written and an intervention designed appropriate to the new objective.

The example in Figure 3.1 is for Scott, the case described in some detail in the previous chapter. An intervention to address work completion in school is presented in greatest detail, while intervention strategies to address impulsivity and homework issues are also presented.

In the real world not all intervention planning is as detailed or precise as we have described here, nor does it need to be. Problems such as forgetting homework materials at school, arriving late for class, or speaking before raising one's hand may be amenable to relatively simple solutions. The guiding principle in designing an intervention should be the least amount of support/training necessary for the student to successfully manage the current problem and similar related problems as they arise. The latter criterion is important since the goal for the child is not only to solve a specific problem but to transfer and generalize the skill to other problems.

Student Name: _Scott_____   Date: _10/4/02_____

I. Data Sources—check all that apply

√ Parent Interview	√ Parent Checklists	√ Classroom Observation
√ Teacher Interview	√ Teacher Checklists	___ Work Samples
___ Student Interview	___ Student Checklists	√ Formal Assessment

II. Areas of Need—fill in applicable sections

Response Inhibition (RI): The capacity to think before acting
Specific problem behaviors (e.g., talks out in class; interrupts; says things without thinking)
1. Talks out in class.
2. Unwanted physical contact with peers.
3.
Working Memory (WM): The ability to hold information in memory while performing complex tasks
Specific problem behaviors (e.g., forgets directions; leaves homework at home; can't do mental arithmetic)
1. Forgets to do homework unless prompted.
2.
3.
Self-Regulation of Affect (SRA): The ability to manage emotions in order to achieve goals, complete tasks, or control or direct behavior
Specific problem behaviors (e.g., "freezes" on tests; gets frustrated when makes mistakes; stops trying in the face of challenge)
1. Overwhelmed by large assignments (whines, complains).
2.
3.
Sustained Attention (SA): The capacity to maintain attention to a situation or task in spite of distractibility, fatigue, or boredom
Specific problem behaviors (e.g., fails to complete classwork on time; stops work before finishing)
1.
2.
3.
Task Initiation (TI): The ability to begin projects without undue procrastination, in an efficient or timely fashion
Specific problem behaviors (e.g., needs cues to start work; puts off long-term assignments)
1. Starts tasks at last minute.
2.
3.

(continued)

FIGURE 3.1. Executive skills: Planning interventions.

FIGURE 3.1. *(page 2 of 6)*

Planning/Prioritization (P): The ability to create a roadmap to reach a goal or to complete a task

Specific problem behaviors (e.g., doesn't know where to start an assignment; can't develop a timeline for long-term assignments)

  1.
  2.
  3.

Organization (O): The ability to arrange or place things according to a system

Specific problem behaviors (e.g., doesn't write down assignments; loses books or papers)

  1.
  2.
  3.

Time Management (TM): The capacity to estimate how much time one has, how to allocate it, and how to stay within time limits and deadlines

Specific problem behaviors (e.g., doesn't work efficiently; can't estimate how long it takes to do something)

  1.
  2.
  3.

Goal-Directed Persistence (GDP): The capacity to have a goal, follow through to the completion of the goal, and not be put off by or distracted by competing interests

Specific problem behaviors (e.g., doesn't see connection between homework and long-term goals; doesn't follow through to achieve stated goals)

  1.
  2.
  3.

Flexibility (F): The ability to revise plans in the face of obstacles, setbacks, new information, or mistakes; it relates to an adaptability to changing conditions

Specific problem behaviors (e.g., gets stuck on one problem-solving strategy; gets upset by unexpected changes to schedule or plans)

  1.
  2.
  3.

Metacognition (M): The ability to stand back and take a bird's-eye view of oneself in a situation; the ability to self-monitor and self-evaluate

Specific problem behaviors (e.g., doesn't have effective study strategies; difficulty catching or correcting mistakes)

  1. *Makes mistakes; doesn't check work.*
  2.
  3.

(continued)

29

FIGURE 3.1. *(page 3 of 6)*

III. Establish Goal Behavior—select specific skill to work on

Target Executive Skill: <u>Working memory, task initiation</u>

Specific Behavioral Objective: <u>Scott will write and follow a daily classwork schedule, as demonstrated by</u> <u>completing 90% of daily assigned tasks with no more than two adult verbal prompts.</u>

IV. Design Intervention

What environmental supports or modifications will be provided to help reach the target goal? *Presentation of brief tasks; alternate nonpreferred with preferred activities; closed-ended tasks (at least at first).*
What specific skills will be taught, who will teach skill, and what procedure will be used to teach the skill(s)? **Skill:** *To make and follow a daily classroom work plan.* **Who will teach skill:** *Teacher.* **Procedure:** *Step 1: The teacher arranges to meet with Scott to explain the process.* *Step 2: They decide how often they need to meet and make a plan.* *Step 3: Teacher explains the planning template to Scott.* *Step 4: Teacher walks Scott through the planning template at the agreed-upon times—* • *"Let's look at what you have to do."* • *Make list of the tasks.* • *Estimate how long it will take to do each task.* • *Decide on start time for each task.* • *Decide on breaks or other reinforcers.* *Step 5: Teacher cues start time.* *Step 6: Teacher checks in at 10-minute intervals to make sure he's following the plan.*
What incentives will be used to help motivate the student to use/practice the skill(s)? *Breaks between tasks (with opportunity to move around and/or read for pleasure).* *Every other task is preferred task (e.g., reading).*

(continued)

FIGURE 3.1. (*page 4 of 6*)

V. Evaluate Intervention

Review date: _____

Was the behavioral objective met?   Yes, completely _____   Yes, partially _____   No _____

Assessment of efficacy of intervention components:

Environmental Supports/Modifications
Were they put in place? Yes.
Were they effective? Yes.
Do they need to be continued? Yes.
Plan for fading supports: Don't fade template, but fade teacher questions as process becomes internalized in working memory and incorporate longer in-class tasks and more advanced assignments.

Skill Instruction
Was the instruction implemented? Yes.
What was the outcome? Scott can make and follow plan without step-by-step instruction.
Does the instruction need to be continued? Yes, when new skills are introduced (e.g., when multistep tasks are introduced).
Plan for fading instruction: Current instructional sequence already faded.

Incentives
Were incentives used? Yes.
Were they effective? Yes.
Do they need to be continued? Yes.
Plan for fading incentives: Retain incentives but increase work time between breaks.

Date for next review: _____

III. Establish Goal Behavior—select specific skill to work on

Target Executive Skill: _Response inhibition_____

Specific Behavioral Objective: _Scott will have "safe hands" (will not engage in hugging, pushing, tripping,_ _kicking, punching, pinching, or other forms of unwelcome physical contact) with classmates._____

IV. Design Intervention

What environmental supports or modifications will be provided to help reach the target goal?
When working independently, Scott will select a work space greater than an arm's length away from the work space of another child.

(continued)

FIGURE 3.1. *(page 5 of 6)*

Make sure he is not in proximity to peers with whom physical contact is a high probability (i.e., other children with problems with response inhibition).

Before free-time activities, teacher will cue Scott to use "safe hands."

For any activity requiring physical contact, teacher will define permitted contact for Scott before the activity begins.

What specific skills will be taught, who will teach skill, and what procedure will be used to teach the skill(s)?

Skill: To use safe hands.

Who will teach skill: Teacher.

Procedure:

Step 1: Explain the skill being worked on ("safe hands"). Give alternative things to do with hands (e.g., fidget toys or a directed activity) when Scott is in situations where problems are likely to arise.
Step 2: Model the skill.
Step 3: Practice the skill, with constructive feedback.
Step 4: Bring in other children to help practice the skill.
Step 5: Cue him to use the skill in classroom and free-time situations.

What incentives will be used to help motivate the student to use/practice the skill(s)?

Verbal feedback; verbal praise.
The alternate activities themselves will be rewarding.
Checks or tokens if necessary.

III. Establish Goal Behavior—select specific skill to work on

Target Executive Skill: Response working memory, task initiation

Specific Behavioral Objective: Scott will write and follow a daily homework schedule, as demonstrated by completing 90% of daily assigned homework with no more than two adult verbal prompts.

IV. Design Intervention

What environmental supports or modifications will be provided to help reach the target goal?

Daily Homework Planner
Adult prompts to make sure homework plan is made and to cue start time(s)

What specific skills will be taught, who will teach skill, and what procedure will be used to teach the skill(s)?

Skill: To make and follow a daily homework plan.

Who will teach skill: Parent/Teacher.

(continued)

FIGURE 3.1. *(page 6 of 6)*

Procedure:

Step 1: Arrange meeting with teacher, parent, and Scott to explain homework process to Scott.

Step 2: Decide on a set time to make the daily plan.

Step 3: Follow planning process—

- "Let's look at what you have for homework."

- Make list of homework tasks.

- Estimate how long it will take to do each task.

- Decide on start time for each task.

- Decide on breaks or other reinforcers.

Step 4: Parent cues start time.

What incentives will be used to help motivate the student to use/practice the skill(s)?

Breaks between tasks.

Fun activity to play when homework is finished.

4

Interventions to Promote Executive Skills

Before we describe interventions to enhance executive skills in children, let's go back and review briefly the developmental nature of these skills. As described in Chapter 1, executive skills are nascent at birth, begin to develop in early infancy, and continue to develop throughout childhood and up to the end of the second decade of life. Some of the more advanced executive skills do not even begin to emerge until age 6 or so, but the reader will do well to remember that, in early development, any of the skills tend to be rudimentary and imperfect, exhibiting themselves inconsistently. Thus, one cannot assume that if we see a very young child restrain herself from performing an illicit act (e.g., taking an unguarded cookie when told cookies are only for dessert), she has the ability to inhibit her behavior at all times and under any circumstance.

In the early stages, it is the job of parents to act as their children's frontal lobes. Thus, in effect, executive skills in very young children are first experienced as external to the child—presented as guidelines or limits by parents or other adults in whose charge they are placed. Gradually, children develop and fine-tune these skills, first by mimicking the executive functions of the adults they observe and eventually by making more independent decisions and choices to regulate their own behavior in the absence of adults.

This gives us the first key principle when thinking about how to help children develop executive skills. *The developmental progression is from external to internal.* When parents or teachers attempt to teach executive skills, they follow this same progression: present them externally first and then—very gradually and potentially over a long time depending on the complexity of the skill being taught and the degree of deficit in the child—fade the instruction, supervision, and cues to the point where the child can apply the skill independently.

A second key principle in developing interventions for children with executive skill deficits also fits this developmental progression from external to internal. Children with underdeveloped executive skills can be supported in one of two ways: (1) by intervening at the level of the environment, or (2) by intervening at the level of the person.

Adults modify the environment by presenting supports, controls, schedules, and other things to reduce the necessity for the child to use executive skills. With a toddler, for instance, we put gates at the head and foot of stairs so the child does not have to decide whether it's safe to climb up or down. We keep food we don't want eaten out of sight or out of reach. We choose clothes appropriate to the weather or the occasion for preschoolers rather than requiring them to make these judgments. And with kindergartners, we're no more likely to send them on a five-step errand than we are to hand them a list of things to do and ask them to read it.

For children with weak executive skills, therefore, the first step is to think about ways to change the environment to adjust to their limitations. While this is often quite effective, the repertoire of interventions cannot stop here; otherwise children would continue to be impaired in their ability to negotiate their world independently. So a second set of interventions involve changing children's skills by teaching them—or motivating them—to develop and use their own executive skills to perform tasks and accomplish goals. When we teach children a procedure to follow to clean their bedrooms, get ready for school in the morning, or get ready to go to bed at night, we are giving them a process they can use on their own eventually in the absence of adult cuing or supervision and across different situations.

As children age, the world demands a greater internalization of executive skills. To the extent that children do not require cuing from adults or environmental supports, they are able to move across environments successfully. This ability to move into new environments successfully is important for parents and teachers to understand because (1) it underscores the importance of generalization (i.e., the ability to take something learned in one situation and apply it in another); (2) it explains why youngsters with severe executive skill deficits are so impaired: they can only operate successfully in settings where the modifications are embedded in the environment rather than presumed to reside within the child.

This chapter will begin by expanding on these two broad domains—intervening at the level of the environment and intervening at the level of the person. We will outline a set of tools that the teacher, parent, or psychologist can draw on to help youngsters with weak executive skills function more effectively. We will then discuss each executive skill in turn and describe ways children can be helped to develop that specific skill.

STRATEGY 1: INTERVENE AT THE LEVEL OF THE ENVIRONMENT

When we talk about intervening at the level of the environment, we mean changing conditions or situations external to the child to improve executive functioning or to reduce the negative effects of weak executive skills. Changing the environment may include (1) changing the physical or social environment to reduce problems; (2) changing the nature of the tasks we expect children to perform; (3) changing the way cues are provided to prompt the child to perform tasks or behave in a certain way; or (4) changing the way people—particularly parents, teachers, and caregivers—interact with children with executive skill deficits.

Changing the Physical or Social Environment

When one is working with children with executive skill deficits, the first step is to survey the physical and social environment in which the child is placed and determine if there are impediments to smooth executive functioning that can be removed or, conversely, if there are things that can be *added to* the environment to enhance functioning. Let's take a child with difficulty sustaining attention by way of example. In a classroom environment, just where that child sits in the classroom can have a significant effect on his or her ability to attend. Children who sit in the back of the classroom, next to a window or an open door, or near their friends or talkative students are likely to have a much more difficult time sustaining attention than are children sitting near the teacher or away from competing distractions. Another example of environmental modification would be to place a child with weak time management or planning/organizational skills with a classroom teacher who's highly structured and adept at helping children plan and use their time well. Finally, children who are inflexible, have a weak ability to inhibit impulses, or have difficulty regulating their affect, are likely to do better in social environments in which the number of children with whom they have to interact is reduced and the degree of adult supervision is increased.

Changing the Nature of the Task

With regard to changing the nature of the tasks we expect children to perform, there are a variety of modifications that can be built into tasks to reduce problems. Table 4.1 outlines some ways that tasks can be modified to help children with executive skill weaknesses be more successful.

We offer the following general rule of thumb regarding task modification. Academic tasks need to be modified so that the *type* and/or *level* of executive skill demand does not exceed the skills of the student to the extent that he or she needs help more than 25% of the time to successfully complete the task. The modifications are less likely to relate to content change and more likely to relate to a change in format (e.g., length, types of directions, mode of response). At this point we are only in the early stages of understanding and assessing the executive skill demands of tasks and hence will need to develop a body of information regarding successful modification of executive demands.

Changing the Way Cues Are Provided

Another way to alter the environment for children with weak executive skills is to build in cues to remind them of the task to be done or the behavior to be performed. Table 4.2 gives examples of such cues.

TABLE 4.1. Altering Tasks to Enhance Success

- *Make the task shorter*, either by reducing the amount of work required or breaking it into pieces with breaks built in along the way.

- *Make the steps more explicit.* The assignment, *Write a paragraph about . . .* , may work for some children, but for those with executive skill deficits, additional structure and guidance will be necessary. This might include spelling out the steps to analyze and solve math word problems, providing "cheat sheets" or templates.

- *Make the task closed ended.* Open-ended tasks can be overwhelming for youngsters with executive skill deficits. They require too much planning, too many choices, or simply too much time to complete. Ways to make tasks closed ended include using fill-in-the-blank or true/false tests rather than essay tests, providing word banks for fill-in-the-blank tests, or allowing children to practice spelling words with magnetic letters rather than using them in sentences.

- *Build in variety or choice* with respect to the tasks to be done or the order in which the tasks are to be done. Have the child suggest ways to alter tasks to make them more interesting or more manageable, or let the child have some say about the order in which the day's work will be completed. This can apply both at home and at school. Teachers might sit down with children at the beginning of the school day to make a daily schedule. Parents, too, often make a homework or chores schedule that gives the child choices.

- *Provide scoring rubrics* to define exactly what is to be included in class assignments. Parents can also apply this principle to home responsibilities by telling their child, "I will know your room is clean when the dirty clothes are put in the laundry, when the clean clothes are in your dresser or closet, when your toys are in your toybox, and when your books are in the bookcase." Better yet, these "steps to a clean room" can be written down in checklist form.

Changing the Way Adults Interact with Students

Finally, for students with executive skill deficits, changing the way adults interact with them can often help ameliorate the negative impact of weak skills. Particularly with younger children, increasing the level of supervision, support, and cuing is the easiest way to impact executive functioning. Table 4.3 lists the advantages of having adults available to cue children.

When adults are used to supervise, support, or cue, we believe this works best when children are involved in the decision-making process and have some role in choosing what role the adult will play and how he or she will play it. This may include having the youngster help decide what cuing system will be used and what incentives will be available to reward the youngster for responding to the cues. This is another way of ensuring a goodness of fit between the youngster and the environment.

While inadequate adult support and supervision leads to obvious problems, over-reliance on adults assuming the role of the child's frontal lobes also has its drawbacks. Although environmental modifications, including adult support, are important tools that can help children with weak executive skills function successfully, the ultimate goal should be to help children develop their own executive skills sufficiently so they can function independently.

TABLE 4.2. Examples of Cues to Prompt Behavior

- *Verbal prompts or reminders.* A teacher might say, "Children coming to the reading group should bring with them the reading book, their workbook, and a pencil." Or a parent might say before a child leaves the house in the morning, "Did you remember to pack your lunch, your gym clothes, and the field trip permission form I signed?"

- *Visual cues.* These can be any kind of posted reminder. Many teachers post the class rules in prominent places in the classroom. The best teachers review those rules regularly, particularly in the beginning of the school year, to help the class remember them.

- *Schedules.* Create a schedule for the child, either for a specific event or for a block of time, such as across a morning or across a school day. For younger children, picture schedules are appropriate; lists or calendar schedules are appropriate for older children. Schedules create an organizational framework and predictability for the child, with the expectation that the schedule will eventually become internalized.

- *Lists.* The content of lists may be things to be remembered (e.g., what to take home from school at the end of the day) or steps to be followed (e.g., how to save a computer file). Children with executive skill deficits are often reluctant to make lists (it's too effortful, takes too much time, or they're very sure they'll remember without having to write anything down). These children need to be encouraged or required to make lists, and in the beginning it's often helpful if someone else makes the list for them and then with them. They may also need secondary cuing systems (i.e., cues to remind them to look at their lists).

- *Audiotaped cues.* One example of an audio cue is a commercially available self-monitoring audiotape designed for children who have difficulty sustaining attention. The tape sounds electronic tones at random intervals, and when the tone sounds the child is instructed to answer the question, "Was I paying attention?" This can be used with a checklist on which she records her answer. Another kind of tape cue are reminder tapes, with verbal messages such as reminders to pay attention, work carefully or slowly, or check work.

- *Pager systems.* This method is particularly appropriate for teenagers since many own pagers or cell phones. Parents can page or call children to remind them to perform some task after school, for instance. A variation on this is a watch with an alarm—or, even better, multiple alarms—that can be set to cue the youngster to remember to do something.

TABLE 4.3. Advantages of Using Adults to Cue Children with Executive Skill Problems

- Problems can be anticipated and the environment altered to avoid them.
- Steps can be taken to intervene early so that a small problem doesn't become a big problem.
- Reminders can be used to prompt children so they avoid the frustration that accompanies forgetting and to increase the likelihood that they perform tasks successfully.
- Situations can be task analyzed through observation, allowing for an improved understanding of the child's skill deficits as well as triggering events that can then facilitate the design of an intervention specific to the child's needs.

STRATEGY 2: INTERVENE AT THE LEVEL OF THE PERSON

The goal of this strategy, broadly speaking, is to change the child's capacity for using her own executive skills. This can be done in one of two ways: (1) by motivating her to use executive skills she has but is reluctant to employ, or (2) by teaching her ways to develop or fine-tune executive skills she needs. In our experience, most youngsters who fail to use executive skills do so not because they don't care but because they don't yet have the executive skill. Thus, we generally recommend that parents and teachers assume this is true and begin tackling executive skill development by teaching the desired skills. However, in many cases interventions at the level of the child involve a combination of both these approaches. This is because learning to use executive skills is often difficult for children with weak executive skills and the addition of an incentive makes practicing the new skills more attractive to the child.

Executive skills are many and varied, and instructional strategies will, by necessity, differ depending on the skill being taught, the context in which it will be used, and the age or developmental level of the child. A general process for teaching children executive skills is outlined in Table 4.4.

By way of example, let's apply this process to a common problem situation in the home: the child who does not clean his or her room. For a very young child or for a child with weak executive skills the directive by a parent to "Go clean your room" produces a response in the child that is inadequate to achieving the desired goal. This response may look different in different children. Some children continue on with whatever task their engaged in, ignoring the parents' request, while others say, "I'll do it later," and then never do it. Still others complain bitterly or throw temper tantrums. Some children may actually go to their bedrooms and begin the task of room cleaning but get distracted or lose interest before the task is done.

So how do parents who want their child to develop more effective executive skills respond? Initially, they become external frontal lobes for their child. In so doing, they perform the following functions:

- They provide a plan, an organizational scheme, and a specific set of directions.
- They monitor performance.
- They provide encouragement, motivation, and feedback about the success of the approach.
- They problem solve when something doesn't work.
- They determine when the task is completed.

In the parents' mind, the problem behavior is *fails to clean room* and the goal behavior is *cleans room when asked without the need for supervision or prompts along the way to completion*. Initially, parents will need to guide their children through the process by using the following kinds of statements or prompts:

"Let's start now."
"Put your trucks in this box."

TABLE 4.4. Teaching Children Executive Skills

Step 1: Describe the problem behaviors.

Examples of problem behaviors might be starting chores but not finishing them, not following morning routines on school days, forgetting to hand in homework assignments, or losing important papers. Be as specific as possible in describing the problem behaviors—they should be described as behaviors that can be seen or heard: "complains about chores" or "rushes through homework, making many mistakes" are better descriptors than "has a bad attitude" or "is lazy."

Step 2: Set a goal

Usually the goal relates directly to the problem behavior. For instance, if not bringing home necessary homework materials is the problem, the goal might be "Mary will bring home from school all necessary materials to complete homework."

Step 3: Establish a procedure or set of steps to reach the goal.

This is usually done best by creating a checklist that outlines the procedure to be followed. See the Appendix for examples of checklists that can be used to address a number of common problems associated with executive skill weaknesses in both home and school settings.

Step 4: Supervise the child following the procedure.

In the early stages, the child will need to be walked through the entire process. Steps include (1) reminding the child to begin the procedure, (2) prompting the child to perform each step in the procedure, (3) observing the child as each step is performed, (4) providing feedback to help improve performance, and (5) praising the child as each step is completed successfully and when the entire procedure is finished.

Step 5: Evaluate the process and make changes if necessary.

At this step, the adult continues to monitor the child's performance to identify where the process might be breaking down or where it might be improved. Most commonly, this will involve tightening the process to include more cues or a more refined breakdown of the task into subtasks. When possible, involve the child in the evaluation process to tap into her problem-solving skills.

Step 6: Fade the supervision.

Decrease the number of prompts and level of supervision to the point where the child is able to follow the procedure independently. This should be done gradually, for example, by (1) prompting the child at each step but leaving the vicinity between steps; (2) getting the child started and making sure she finishes but not being present while she performs the task; (3) cuing the child to start, to use the checklist to check off as each step is completed, and to report back when done; and (4) prompting the child to "use your checklist" with no additional cues or reminders. Ultimately, the child will either retrieve the checklist on her own or even be able to perform the task without the need for a checklist at all.

"Put your dirty clothes in the laundry."

"Put your books on the bookshelf."

"There are two toys under the bed you missed."

"It doesn't look like all those toys will fit in that one box; we'll need to get another box (choose some toys to put in the attic)."

"When you finish, you can play with your friends."

"I know you hate doing this now, but you'll feel so much better when it's done."

"There, doesn't that feel great now that you've got a clean room? And your work is over for the day!"

After having walked the child through the process many times, parents can begin to reduce the level of support and supervision. They might, for instance, provide the same information without being the direct agent. Ways to do this include creating a list, picture cues, an audiotape, and the like to cue the child. In this case, the parent might say to the child, "Look at your list." The next step might be to begin to transfer the responsibility to the child by asking a more general question (e.g., "What do you need to do?"). The transfer is complete when the child reaches the point where he asks himself, "What do I need to do?" and either refers to the list independently without prompting from the parent or remembers the steps on the list and can perform the task without referring to the list itself.

In addition to teaching children to use executive skills, a second intervention at the level of the child is to motivate children to use executive skills already within their repertoire. Although punishment or imposing penalties are options when trying to motivate children to change their behavior, we generally espouse a positive approach. For children for whom the acquisition of executive skills comes easily, this positive approach may be as simple as providing praise and recognition whenever children use these skills. A parent might say to their 5-year-old, for instance, "You remembered to brush your teeth after breakfast without my having to remind you. That's great!" Remembering to notice and respond when children engage in appropriate behaviors (whether executive skills or any other desired behavior) can be a powerful way to shape behavior.

When that is not enough, however, parents or teachers may find it helpful to use some kind of incentive system to motivate children to use executive skills. The steps in developing incentive systems are described in Table 4.5.

Figure 4.1 provides an example of how the planning process might work. Figure 4.2 is a sample behavior contract that might be drawn up to address the problem behavior depicted in Figure 4.1. The Appendix contains the forms necessary to design an incentive system and write a behavior contract.

Parents often ask how they can develop this kind of system for one child in the family and not for all children, since it may seem to be "rewarding" children with problems while neglecting those without. We have found that most siblings are understanding of this process if it is explained to them carefully. If there are problems, however, parents have several choices: (1) set up a similar system for other children with appropriate goals (*every* child has *something* he or she could be working to improve); (2) make a more informal arrangement by promising to do something special from time to time with the other children in the family so they don't feel left out; or (3) have the child earn rewards that benefit the whole family (e.g., eating out at a Chinese restaurant).

One important role for parents or teachers to play is to ensure that there are adequate environmental supports in place to help the child be successful. In the example below, an environmental support is a chore list, and it's the parents' role to make sure the support is in place. The next section will give numerous examples of environmental supports that can be used for specific executive skill deficits.

TABLE 4.5. Designing Incentive Systems

Steps 1 and 2: Describe the problem behaviors and set a goal.

These are identical to Steps 1 and 2 for teaching the child to use executive skills (see Table 4.4). Both problem and goal behaviors should be described as specifically as possible, usually with a link between the two. As an example, if forgetting to do chores after school is the problem, the goal might be "Joe will complete daily chores without reminders before 4:30 in the afternoon."

Step 3: Decide on possible rewards and contingencies.

Incentive systems work best when children have a "menu" of rewards to choose from. One of the best ways to do this is a point system in which points can be earned for the goal behaviors and traded in for the reward the child wants to earn. The bigger the reward, the more points the child will need to earn it. The menu should include both larger, more expensive rewards that may take a week or a month to earn, and smaller, inexpensive rewards that can be earned daily. Rewards can include "material" reinforcers (such as favorite foods or small toys) as well as activity rewards (such as the chance to play a game with a parent, teacher, or friend). It may also be necessary to build contingencies into the system—usually the access to a privilege after a task is done (such as the chance to watch a favorite TV show or the chance to talk on the telephone to a friend).

When incentive systems are used in a school setting, it is often beneficial to build in a home component. This is because parents often have available a wider array of reinforcers than are available to teachers. When a coordinated approach is used, a home–school report card is often the vehicle by which teachers communicate to parents how many points the child has earned that day. Situations in which we do not recommend including a home component include (1) when parents, for whatever reason, are unable to maintain the system consistently; (2) when parents insist on negative consequences; or (3) when the child needs a more immediate reward and cannot wait until the end of the school day to earn it.

Once the system is up and running, if you find the child is earning more penalties than rewards, then the program needs to be revised so that the child can be more successful. Usually when this kind of system fails, we think of it as a "design failure" rather than the failure of the child to respond to rewards.

Step 4: Write a behavior contract.

The contract should say exactly what the child agrees to do and exactly what the parents' or teacher's roles and responsibilities will be. Along with points and rewards, parents or teachers should be sure to praise children for following the contract. It will be important for adults to agree to a contract they can live with: they should avoid penalties they are either unable or unwilling to impose (e.g., if both parents work and are not at home, they cannot monitor whether a child is beginning his or her homework right after school, so an alternative contract may need to be written).

Step 5: Evaluate the process and make changes if necessary.

Incentive systems may not work the first time. Parents or teachers should expect to try it out and redesign it to work the kinks out. Eventually, once the child is used to doing the behaviors specified in the contract, the contract can be rewritten to work on another problem behavior. As time goes on, children may be willing to drop the use of an incentive system altogether. This is often a long-term goal, however, and adults should be ready to write a new contract if the child slips back to bad habits once a system is dropped.

INCENTIVE PLANNING SHEET

Problem Behavior
Forgetting to do chores after school.

Goal
Complete chores by 4:30 P.M. without reminders.

Possible Rewards

Daily	Weekly	Long-Term
Extra TV show.	Chance to rent video game.	Buy video game.
Extra video game time.	Have friend spend night on weekend.	Buy CD.
Play game with Dad.	Mom will make favorite dessert.	Go skiing.
Extra half-hour before bed.	Chance to choose dinner menu.	Eat out.

Possible Contingencies
Can play with friends after school as soon as chores are done.
Access to TV/video games after chores are done.

FIGURE 4.1. Planning an incentive system.

SAMPLE BEHAVIOR CONTRACT

Student agrees to complete chores by 4:30 P.M. without verbal reminders.

To help student reach goal, parents will place a chore list on kitchen table before child comes home from school.

Student will earn five points for each day he completes chores without verbal reminders. Points can be traded in for items on the reward menu.

If student fails to meet agreement, student will not earn any points.

FIGURE 4.2. Sample contract.

HOME–SCHOOL COLLABORATION

Embedded in the notions of environmental support and teaching the child improved executive skills is the assumption that key adults (i.e., parents and teachers) are available and willing to lend their efforts—and frontal lobes—to this task. Experience tells us that this is not always the case. Parents, for example, may have executive skill challenges similar to those of their children, reflecting the proverbial short distance between apple and tree. Or the parent(s) simply may not have the resources or see that the cost of such an effort is exceeded by the benefits. Teachers often already feel overwhelmed by the demands of their jobs, and each new request adds one more straw. They also may see the issue as a motivational deficit rather than a skill deficit and hence frame it as the child's problem to solve. Whatever the reason, the fact remains that a supportive adult is necessary for the success of the intervention. If initial adult support is not available in one or the other setting, we offer the following considerations.

Parental Support Unavailable

When parent support is requested for a school-based executive problem, it is typically around some aspect of homework. Parents may not have the time or organizational skills to manage this, or conflict between parent and child around this issue may preclude their help. When a parent is unavailable, there are two options. One is to move the homework piece into the school, using study periods and/or an after-school homework club. We also have been able to use after-school child-care programs by providing an incentive to the child for homework completion. A second option is to use a coach (see Chapter 5). This has been quite effective at middle and high school levels where students often resent parent efforts to monitor homework and other school responsibilities.

Teacher Support Unavailable

When a teacher feels that he or she cannot provide the support necessary, there are a few options. If in-class cuing and support is needed, then rather than intervening all day long, one time during the day when the executive skill weakness is most evident can be selected (e.g., circle time; independent work). Another adult such as a school counselor, teacher aide, or speech pathologist could provide the support during this limited time. When carried out in conjunction with a daily incentive system for the child, a skill can be rapidly acquired. With this success, the teacher may be encouraged to provide cuing in other situations to promote generalization, or the adult who provided the original help may come in at a new time. Another option is to use a classmate or an older student as an in-class mentor. One school we work with uses eighth-grade students to help sixth graders with organization and time management. A school counselor or psychologist may also be able to provide a teacher with high- or low-tech solutions (e.g., cuing/signaling devices) to decrease the labor intensity of the support needed. As noted above, coaching with another adult in school also offers an option to support executive skills without adding to the workload of the teacher.

Successful interventions with executive skills are possible, in our experience, even when adult support in one area may not be optimal. Still, chances for success are best when parents and teachers can work collaboratively with the child to first provide and then gradually fade the supports needed to develop executive skills.

INTERVENTIONS FOR SPECIFIC EXECUTIVE SKILL DEFICITS

Now we turn to interventions designed to enhance specific executive skills. These interventions have been "field tested," and we are satisfied, based on parent and teacher feedback, that they fit well with real-world demands. Nonetheless, keep in mind that the suggestions provided will not work with all children and that adaptations will need to be made particularly with respect to the developmental level of the child or the severity of the problem.

As a general metaphor to help readers understand the process of enhancing executive skills, think of these tools as ways to assist children on a journey. The kinds of modifications and strategies we describe below can be thought of as ways to shorten the journey, help travelers see their destination more clearly, give them signposts to let them know they're on the right road and to mark their progress, give them a "roadmap" to guide them—or maybe even a Global Positioning System spelling out more precisely where they are and where they need to go next.

Think for a moment about the concept of a roadmap. A roadmap provides directions for how to get from a starting point to an ending point. If I don't know how to get some place, I have someone draw me a map. In the beginning, I need to bring that map with me and refer to it frequently so I don't get lost. But if I go to that same place often enough, I no longer need the map. This is because I've *internalized* the map and can rely on my own mental representation of the directions to get me where I need to go. This same approach applies to improving executive skills. Initially, we draw children a map and we prompt them to refer to the map so they don't get lost. With practice, they no longer need either the map or the external cues to use because they have internalized it and can follow the procedure on their own.

The remainder of this chapter will present one table for each executive skill (Tables 4.6 to 4.16). Each table will include the following components: (1) suggested environmental modifications that can be put in place for the youngster with a weakness in that executive skill area, (2) examples of steps or procedures that can be followed to teach the skill, and (3) a brief vignette that illustrates an application of environmental modifications or skill instruction to a typical home or school situation in which the executive skill might be displayed.

We need to caution readers not to look at what follows as a "cookbook" designed to produce solutions to very specific problems. Rather, we hope that readers recognize that executive skill deficits will incur problems that arise *across* situations. For instance, youngsters with time management problems generally don't just have problems managing their time in order to complete schoolwork; they generally also have difficulty managing their time in other arenas—completing chores, getting to appointments on time, deciding how they are going to spend their free time, etc. As you read through the following section, we encourage you to consider executive skill weakness more broadly and how it comes into play in specific situations in a youngster's daily life.

We also should note that while each executive skill has unique aspects to it, there are common interventions that apply across executive skills in some cases. For this reason, some interventions will be mentioned in more than one table, or the reader will be referred to related skills for additional suggestions.

TABLE 4.6. Response Inhibition

Description of skill

The capacity to think before you act; the capacity to delay or inhibit responding based on the ability to evaluate multiple factors. Children who have trouble with response inhibition are impulsive, saying or doing things without thinking, which often gets them into trouble with parents, teachers, or peers.

Environmental modifications

- Increase external controls—in other words, restrict access to settings or situations in which the child can get in trouble. A child who may run out into the road to retrieve a ball is not allowed to play in the front yard or not allowed to play outdoors without supervision. If a child throws things in anger, parents keep expensive or breakable objects out of reach.
- Increase supervision. When parents say, "I can't let him out of my sight," this suggests they have modified the environment by making sure there is an adult present at all times to reduce the likelihood that the child will do something dangerous or forbidden. Children with impulse control problems, particularly when they are young, often require more adult supervision in school settings. This is why the adult-to-student ratio is greater in preschools than in middle school. It is also why schools will sometimes assign individual aides to children. The physical presence of an adult in proximity to the child with impulse control problems acts as a cue for the child to exercise control.
- Find ways to cue the child to control impulses. This may include posting and reviewing class rules or stopping a child before she goes out to recess to ask, "What behavior are we working on?" to remind the child to exhibit self-control in specific situations (the child might say in answer to that question, "Not hitting when I get mad").

Teaching the skill

Focus of instruction: to teach the child a competing skill to replace the disinhibited response. For instance, if blurting out in class is the problem, then teach the child to raise her hand before speaking.

Steps to follow:
1. Explain to the child the skill being worked on and your understanding of the intent of the child's behavior (e.g., "I think you talk out because you're looking for recognition from me or your classmates. We're going to work on raising your hand before you speak"). In selecting the replacement skill (e.g., hand raising), make sure the skill being taught meets the same need (i.e., peer or teacher recognition).
2. Walk the child through the process, having her practice the skills using a contrived situation or a teaching example. Practice the skill sufficiently so that the child can be successful most of the time (you may want to make a game of the process, such as a variation of *Simon Says*). For instance, if hand raising is the skill being taught, then the practice could include keeping score for how many times the child remembers to raise her hand before speaking during the practice sessions.
3. At the point when the child is ready to use the skill in the natural environment, the child should be cued to use the skill just prior to the situation in which the skill will be required (e.g., by saying to the child, "Remember what we're working on").
4. Reinforce the child immediately for using the skill (e.g., if hand raising is the skill being taught, then early in the training stage, call on the child right away whenever she raises her hand and praise her for remembering to raise her hand).
5. Ignore the disinhibited response (e.g., don't respond when she blurts out).
6. Gradually fade the cuing and reinforcement (e.g., by not calling on her right away every time she raises her hand). This may be even more effective if you tell the child that this is what you are going to do (e.g., "I'm not going to call on you every time. I won't forget you're there, but I'm only going to call on you every fourth or fifth time.").

(continued)

TABLE 4.6. (continued)

Vignette

Circle time was a constant struggle for Kristin and her teacher, Mrs. Brock. In spite of rules about turn taking and not interrupting every day, Kristin would blurt out information when someone else was talking instead of raising her hand and waiting to be called on. Mrs. Brock decided that providing some cues and a plan for Kristin could help. She first introduced a "talking stick" to the class and indicated that only the person who had the stick could speak at that moment. She also gave two chips to each child that they could "spend" by asking two questions once the speaker indicated it was time for questions. At this point, the children would raise their hands and the teacher would call on one. Recognizing Kristin's difficulty waiting, for the first week the teacher called on her first. If Kristin forgot and blurted something out before the speaker was finished, she had to give up one of her chips. This, along with initially sitting next to the teacher, was usually sufficient to help her remember. However, on a few occasions Kristin (and a few other children) "spent" both chips before the speaker was done and needed to leave the circle. Kristin found this system helpful, and after the first week she was able to decide with her teacher how many children she felt she could wait for before asking her questions.

TABLE 4.7. Working Memory

<u>Description of skill</u>

The ability to hold information in mind while performing complex tasks. It incorporates the ability to draw on past learning or experience to apply to the situation at hand or to project into the future.

<u>Environmental modifications</u>

These are usually either storage mechanisms or cuing mechanisms, designed to help the child store information in memory (or in some other more readily retrievable location, such as a calendar or notebook) or to cue the child to retrieve the information on demand or at a set time.

Storage devices include the following:
- Agenda books or calendars (e.g., for writing down assignments or appointments).
- Notebooks (e.g., for keeping to-do lists).
- Electronic devices such as Palm Pilots, tape recorders, or message systems (e.g., some people call their answering machines to remind them of things they need to do when they get home; others use electronic messaging devices).

Cuing devices include the following:
- Arranging for verbal reminders (e.g., from parent, teacher, aide, or peer).
- Page systems.
- Alarms on watches (some watches allow for multiple alarms).
- Visual cues displayed in a prominent place (writing on the back of one's hand; Post-it software for the computer desktop; etc.).
- Taking advantage of a naturally occurring cue in the environment. This can be manipulated by placing the cue in a prominent place where it's not likely to be missed. For example, if a child has trouble remembering to take morning medication, she could place the pill bottle directly in front of the box of cereal on the breakfast table. Another example would be to incorporate recurring phrases teachers might use or teacher behaviors (e.g., using the music's teacher's tapping his baton on the desk to bring the class to order as a signal to a child to stop talking).

For cues to be effective, they should ideally be unusual or unexpected so that they do not blend into their surroundings. Auditory cues tend to be more effective than visual ones, because they're more likely to cause the individual to attend to the cue (if only to ask, "What's *that*?"). It's also possible to increase the salience of the cue by having the child practice responding to it.

<u>Teaching the skill</u>

Rather than assigning cues, teach the child to design his or her own cues and to put systems in place to use the cues. The steps to follow are:
1. Explain the problem as it shows in the child.
2. With younger children, give them a range of options and have them pick one that's appealing. Or have them generate their own.
3. Mentally rehearse the association between the cue and the working memory. Then use in vivo rehearsal.
4. Devise a monitoring system (e.g., Did you use the cue? Yes/No. How well did you do?).

<u>Vignette</u>

Mario, age 11, was continually forgetting things he needed to bring home from school, such as his homework, his assignment book, and permission slips to be signed. His mother kept having to drive him back to school to collect the things he forgot. She did this for a while, then she felt she was rewarding him for forgetting, so she stopped. Sometimes he would earn a lower grade on his homework or he would have to serve a detention for forgetting assignments, but this didn't seem to help him remember. His mother met with his teacher to see if there might be a better way to handle the problem. Together, Mario's mother and teacher and Mario himself developed a list of the things he might need to remember to bring home each day. His teacher added some things he tended to forget to do during the school day as well (see Getting Ready to Go Home *in the Appendix). They placed the checklist in a plastic sleeve and had Mario use a pen that could be erased after he completed the checklist each day. During the last 10 minutes of the school day, a teacher aide and Mario went through the checklist item by item. For quite a while, the aide needed to stay with Mario to make sure he completed the entire checklist. Eventually, she was able just to prompt Mario to "get out your checklist" and to check with him after he'd completed it.*

TABLE 4.8. Self-Regulation of Affect

Description of skill

The ability to manage emotions in order to achieve goals, complete tasks, or control and direct behavior.

Environmental modifications

These are designed to help students manage their emotions (both positive and negative) more effectively. They include the following:

- Anticipating problem situations and preparing child for them.
- Teaching coping strategies. For example, children who get anxious before exams can learn relaxation techniques.
- Giving children scripts to follow in target situations, or things they can say to themselves to help them manage emotions.
- Structuring the environment to avoid problem situations or to intervene early. For example, if children become overstimulated in social situations, then limit the number of children they play with or increase the structure of the play activity.
- Breaking tasks into smaller steps to make them more manageable.
- Giving the child a break if a task appears to be becoming upsetting.
- Having adults model the practice of making positive self-statements. For instance, a parent or teacher might say to the child, "Here's what I want you to say to yourself before starting this: 'I know this will be hard for me, but I'm going to keep trying. If I get stuck after trying hard, I will ask for help.'"
- Giving "pep talks" to the child before beginning a task.
- Teaching the child that how you think about an experience can affect how you feel about that experience. Examples from sports psychology for older children or superheroes for younger children may be a good way to do this.
- Using literature (such as *The Little Engine That Could*) or writing individualized social stories to teach emotional control.

Teaching the skill

This involves teaching the child to independently use strategies such as those described above. For example, the child could be taught to identify and use a coping strategy when she encounters a problem situation or the child could be taught to use other strategies such as breaking a task down, creating a script, or making positive self-statements. A general outline for teaching this kind of skill is:

1. Explain the skill to the child.
2. Have the child practice the skill.
3. Reinforce the child for practicing well.
4. Cue the child to use the skill in real-life situations (classroom or home settings).
5. Reinforce the child for using the skill successfully.

Specific strategies that children can be taught to use include:

- Self-statements to promote a positive emotional response or an effective coping strategy.
- Having the child verbalize a goal behavior ("Today I will _____") before entering the situation where she can display the goal behavior.
- The use of visual imagery. Here, teach the child to visualize himself managing the problem situation successfully. For example, if the child tends to be a poor sport on the athletic field, have him picture the umpire calling him out on a questionable strike and then have him picture himself walking back to the dugout with a calm expression on his face.
- Having the child incorporate practicing the skill into something she does routinely every day (e.g., journal writing at school or a bedtime routine where the child describes a positive use of the skill to a parent who puts her to bed at night).

(continued)

TABLE 4.8. (*continued*)

<u>Vignette</u>

Recess was often a traumatic time for Timmy, age 6. He loved swinging on a particular swing, but it was often in use by someone else when he got out to the playground. Once he got the swing for himself, he resisted giving it up to let someone else swing. The teacher on duty finally decided the best way to handle it was to teach Timmy a strategy for managing his emotions. She made a deal with Timmy that he could swing on the swing for the first 5 minutes of recess and then, if he gave up the swing to another child without a fight, he could swing again for the last 3 minutes of recess. She taught Timmy to say to himself, "If I don't get mad, I can have another turn" as he got off the swing. Before they used this plan at recess, she took Timmy out to the playground on his own to practice getting off the swing and saying the statement about not getting mad. They practiced this several times until Timmy thought he would be able to do it successfully at recess. Both during the practice sessions and once they started following the procedure at recess, his teacher praised him for following the plan successfully. In time, she taught Timmy to wait for a turn at the beginning of recess by saying to himself, "I can wait; it will be my turn soon." Before the year was over, Timmy was even able to invite other children to use his favorite swing and to give up his own turn to let someone else swing.

TABLE 4.9. Sustained Attention

Description of skill

The capacity to maintain attention to a situation or task in spite of distractibility, fatigue, or boredom.

Environmental modifications

These are designed either to accommodate to students' difficulty with sustained attention or to make it easier for them to attend longer to tasks. They might include the following:

- Writing start and stop times on assigned tasks to help students persist with tasks long enough to complete them.
- Using incentive systems. For youngsters who have no interest in the work they're being asked to do, extrinsic rewards are sometimes the best hope for success. To be effective, they need to be powerful, frequent, and varied. Examples include awarding points for completed work or for work completed within specific time parameters, or arranging for a preferred activity to immediately follow less attractive tasks in order to give the student something to look forward to.
- Breaking tasks into subtasks and giving the student short breaks after each subtask.
- Setting a kitchen timer and challenging the student to complete the task within the time allotted.
- Using a self-monitoring tape (an audiotape that sounds electronic tones at random intervals and asking the student to ask himself, "Was I paying attention?" each time the tone sounds.
- Choosing the time of day carefully (e.g., having children do difficult tasks at the time of day when they are most alert).
- Providing supervision. Youngsters attend best in situations in which they receive one-to-one attention, frequent feedback, and immediate reinforcement. Research also suggests that children with problems with sustained attention have less difficulty when working with fathers than when working with mothers. This may have implications for who supervises homework.
- Making tasks interesting for students, since people work longer and harder on tasks of interest to them than on those they consider tedious, boring, or not important. Ways to do this may include making the task active or interactive, or turning the task into a challenge, a game, or a contest.
- Giving the child something to look forward to that can be done as soon as the task is finished (e.g., allowing a seventh grader the chance to "instant message" her friends as soon as her homework is done).
- Providing attention and praise when the student is on task.

Teaching the skill

Teaching children to sustain attention involves teaching them to internalize the externally imposed strategies described above. This can be done by:

1. Helping youngsters become aware of their own attentional capacity (e.g., how long they can work before they need a break).
2. Teaching them how to break a task down into pieces that fit their attentional capacity.
3. Helping them make a work plan. This should include helping them allocate work according to their capacity, but it should also include helping them identify both motivational strategies and environmental cues they can use to help them stay on task. Motivational strategies might include finding ways to make the task more active (e.g., not just *reading* a social studies chapter but posing a question to read for, note taking, creating a graphic organizer, or highlighting) or creating a script to keep them going (the son of one of the authors used to tell himself, "You *can't* walk away from this" when he found his attention flagging during homework). Environmental cues might include setting kitchen timers or alarm clocks, or asking an adult to check in on them periodically to make sure they're working.
4. Cuing them to follow the plan they've devised.
5. Reinforcing them for following the plan successfully.
6. Gradually transferring the responsibility for making the plan to the students themselves.

(continued)

TABLE 4.9. (*continued*)

Vignette

Sarah, a fourth grader, had the hardest time getting her seatwork done. When the teacher assigned a task, she might start it right away, but she would become quickly distracted. She might get up and sharpen her pencil, go to the bathroom, or talk to the other students sitting at her table. Sometimes she might overhear a conversation at the next table and feel like she had to participate in that discussion. Her teacher used to keep her in from recess to finish her work or to send it home for homework, but her parents raised objections to this. So she decided to try a different approach. She sat down with Sarah and explained that getting her work done on time was important. She asked Sarah to think about what makes it hard to get her work done. Sarah was able to generate a long list; she included things like "My pencil lead breaks; other kids' talking distracts me; I get tired; sometimes I don't know how to do the work; I get bored; my hand gets tired of writing." The more they talked, the more it became apparent that the main reasons Sarah wasn't getting work done were because she got distracted and she thought the work was tedious. Her teacher decided it would be good to involve her parents in this, in part because they were resistant to her missing recess and bringing unfinished work home at night. All together they came up with two interventions: (1) Sarah's parents agreed that any day she came home with all her work done, she could watch a favorite daily TV show that she was usually only able to watch on school vacations; (2) Sarah agreed to work on trying to pay attention better. Her teacher brought out the self-monitoring tape and explained how it worked. She combined the tape with a checklist so that whenever the tone sounded, Sarah was to circle Yes or No on the checklist to indicate whether she was paying attention. This was quite successful. After a period of time, the teacher removed the checklist and had Sarah just ask herself whether she was paying attention each time she heard the tone. The third step in fading the intervention was to place a sticker on Sarah's desk to use both as a cue to pay attention and as a reminder for her to ask herself if she was paying attention. Gradually Sarah was able to improve her efficient work production due to better attention.

TABLE 4.10. Task Initiation

Description of skill

The ability to begin a task without undue procrastination, in a timely fashion.

Environmental modifications

These are designed to help children get right to work when tasks are assigned or to begin them at a predetermined time. They include the following:

- Verbally cuing the child to get started.
- Arranging for a visual cue to prompt the child to begin (e.g., a picture taped to the desk).
- Walking the child through the first portion of the task to get them started.
- Noting start and stop times when tasks are assigned/completed.
- Having the child specify when she will begin the task and then cuing her when the scheduled time arrives (this approach can be used quite successfully for homework or chores). Alternatively, have the child decide how she will be cued to begin the task (e.g., by using an alarm clock or a naturally occurring event to act as the cue, such as "immediately after lunch").

Teaching the skill

There are two kinds of task initiation: the first involves beginning a task right away when it is assigned, and the second involves planning when a task will be done and starting it promptly at the predetermined time.

To begin tasks promptly, teach the child either to self-instruct (i.e., talk to herself by saying something like "The teacher told us what to do and now it's time to start") or to perform right away the first step in the assigned task (open the textbook, get out pencil and paper, write her name at the top of the paper, etc.).

Teaching a child to begin a task promptly at some future predetermined time can be done with the following steps:

1. Have the child make a written plan for doing the task. This may include writing down the assignment and deciding on a start time. For longer projects, it may mean breaking the task down into subtasks and assigning start times to each subtask.
2. Have the child determine what cue will be used to remind her to begin the task. This could include having a parent or teacher (or sibling or friend) provide the reminder, setting some kind of alarm, or using a naturally occurring event as the cue.
3. At the point when the child is expected to begin the task, make sure she does so promptly, reinforcing her when she does not require additional cues beyond those she built into the plan.
4. Gradually fade the supervision.

This skill also lends itself to an incentive system to reinforce practicing the skill successfully. The child could earn points, for instance, for starting the task on time, with points redeemable for small rewards.

Vignette

Lisa, age 9, had a very difficult time starting her homework promptly at the time her parents set for her (right after dinner). Her parents decided they needed to teach this as a skill. Every day when she came home from school, her mother sat down with her and they made out a homework plan (see Homework Planning Sheet *in the Appendix). Lisa made a list of all her assignments and she wrote down when she would start each one. She was allowed to build in a break for one TV show. When it was time for her to start her homework, her mother pulled out the Homework Planner and asked Lisa to take a look at it. Lisa then got out the first assignment and her mother made sure she got off to a good start before she left to do other things. In the beginning Lisa's mother praised her for following her schedule and when she completed each activity. As time went on, Lisa was able to make her schedule and follow it all by herself.*

TABLE 4.11. Planning

<u>Description of skill</u>

The ability to create a roadmap to reach a goal or to complete a task. It also involves being able to make decisions about what's important to focus on and what's not important.

<u>Environmental modifications</u>

By modifying the environment, the necessity for the youngster to rely on his own planning skills is reduced. Modifications might include:

- Have the adult provide a plan or a schedule for the child to follow.
- Use scoring rubrics when giving students assignments.
- Break long-term projects into clearly defined subtasks and attach deadlines to each subtask (many teachers incorporate this into their long-term project requirements).
- Create a template (see *Long-Term Project Planning Sheet* in the Appendix).

<u>Teaching the skill</u>

The best way to teach children to plan is to walk them through the planning process many times with multiple kinds of tasks, gradually turning over the process to the youngsters by asking questions that prompt them to think about how to make a plan. In the early stages, the questions will need to prompt each step (What do you have to do first? What do you have to do next?). As youngsters become more experienced with this, the prompts can be more general (e.g., "Okay, let's make a list of all the things you have to do to complete this project"; "Now let's organize those tasks in order in which you need to do them").

Using the analogy of the roadmap may be an effective way to help students think about what planning requires. Using this analogy, have the youngsters identify the destination (or goal). Then have them visualize the path they need to take to reach the destination. With younger children, giving them a planning sheet that actually looks like a roadmap may facilitate the process.

<u>Vignette</u>

Tom, an eighth grader, had a bad habit of leaving projects until the last minute and then having no idea what he had to do to complete the assignment. This created a great deal of tension at home as he experienced meltdowns as deadlines approached. His mother finally decided to intervene. Using a weekly progress report, she arranged with the school to be notified directly when long-term projects were assigned. Then she sat down with Tom to draw up a plan for each assignment using the Long-Term Project Planning Sheet. *The first time they used it, Tom had to write a report on a dangerous sea animal (see Figure 4.3). She helped Tom brainstorm topics and identify all the materials he needed to complete the project. Then they took a calendar and, as they planned each step, wrote down deadlines on the calendar. Then they placed the calendar in a prominent place in the kitchen so Tom could check it easily each day. Since they used a form and calendar to complete the planning process, Tom's mother could gradually turn the process over to him. Eventually, she was able to remind him to do the planning, but he could do the rest on his own.*

STEP 1: SELECT TOPIC

What are possible topics?	What I like about this choice:	What I don't like:
1. Octopus	They have eight legs, and I've always wanted to know how they use them.	Might not be able to find enough material.
2. Giant Squid	I want to know how they make the ink they spray and how they spray it.	There might not be enough other stuff about them that's interesting.
3. Killer whale	I've always been interested in whales, and I have a lot of books on the topic.	I know so much, I might not learn anything new.
4. White shark	They're more deadly to humans than the other things on my list.	At least two other kids in the class are choosing this topic.
5.		

Final Topic Choice:

White shark

STEP 2: IDENTIFY NECESSARY MATERIALS

What materials or resources do you need?	Where will you get them?	When will you get them?
1. Encyclopedia (for overview).	School library.	During class.
2. At least 2 books or chapters.	School library/town library.	During class or this Saturday.
3. Pictures.	Internet.	After I've done my research.
4.		
5.		

(continued)

FIGURE 4.3. Long-Term Project Planning Sheet.

56

STEP 3: IDENTIFY PROJECT TASKS AND DUE DATES

What do you need to do? (List each step in order.)	When will you do it?	Check off when done
Step 1: Take notes from encyclopedia.	English class this Friday.	
Step 2: Check books out of library.	English class on Friday (school library) or this Saturday (town library).	
Step 3: Take notes from books.	Mon.–Fri. next week (half hour a day).	
Step 4: Look for pictures on Internet.	Next Saturday.	
Step 5: Organize note cards.	Next Saturday.	
Step 6: Outline report.	Next Sunday.	
Step 7: Write first half of report.	A week from Monday.	
Step 8: Write second half of report.	A week from Tuesday.	
Step 9: Edit/proofread.	A week from Wednesday.	
Step 10: Add pictures; do final touches.	A week from Thursday.	

FIGURE 4.3. (*continued*)

TABLE 4.12. Organization

Description of skill

The ability to arrange or place things according to a system.

Environmental modifications

One basic environmental modification presents itself for this particular executive skill: youngsters who lack organizational capacity need to be given organizational schemes to work with. For this to work successfully, two other components need to be built in: children need to be cued to use the organizational scheme, and they need to be reinforced for doing so. Examples of the kinds of organizational schemes children might be taught to use are:

- Room-cleaning schemes. This can be facilitated by giving children plastic bins labeled for the possessions that are to be stored in each one.
- A system for organizing a backpack, such as specific pockets for lunch, permission slips, or money.
- A system for organizing schoolwork, such as using different colored folders to distinguish completed assignments from work not yet done.
- A system for organizing the student's desk, either at home or at school.

Many parents and teachers are quite adept at creating organizational schemes for youngsters. Where the process breaks down is the degree of supervision required to ensure that the child actually uses the scheme on a day-in, day-out basis. We also recommend adding a powerful reinforcer to ensure that the youngster uses the scheme. We know of a mother of a middle school student who threatened to send to Goodwill any clothes her son left lying on his bedroom floor. Although we generally recommend using positive reinforcement, we have to admit that this was a powerful incentive for this youngster to keep his bedroom clean.

Teaching the skill

For youngsters with genuinely weak organizational skills, teaching this skill is a long-term proposition. For the youngest of children, an important prerequisite is the ability to separate or categorize (see how this is incorporated into the *Desk Cleaning Checklist* in the Appendix). Once youngsters have learned this skill, then we recommend teaching them to become organized by giving them lots of different organizational schemes for different aspects of their lives and having them overlearn those schemes (via cuing, practice, and reinforcement). As they internalize the schemes, the cuing and reinforcement can be faded.

Giving youngsters a variety of organizational systems will provide them with common templates on which they can draw when they begin to develop their own systems. Once they have internalized the schemes provided to them, new tasks can be introduced and they can be asked to hypothesize new organizational schemes to fit those tasks. At first they will need assistance in doing this, but they should be encouraged to look upon the process as a problem to be solved for which creativity may be required. For youngsters with weak organizational skills, working with a coach, as described in Chapter 5, may be an effective intervention.

Vignettes

Josh, a fifth grader, had the messiest desk in his class. He lost papers all the time, and it took him way longer than anyone else to locate his work materials. His teacher, Mr. Carroll, used to let a month go by, then keep him in from recess to get his desk clean. Josh hated missing recess, and his teacher hated nagging him. Finally, Mr. Carroll decided there might be a better way. Although Josh was the worst, there were others in the class that had messy desks too, so Mr. Carroll decided that Friday afternoons would be desk-cleaning time. Those who had clean desks could get a jump start on their homework for the weekend. He brainstormed with the class what steps students need to go through to clean their desks. They created a checklist (see Desk Cleaning Checklist in the Appendix). Now every Friday Mr. Carroll quickly checks each desk and decides who needs to use the checklist to clean their desks.

(continued)

TABLE 4.12. (*continued*)

Joan, a ninth grader, was forever losing worksheets and assignments. She tended to work slowly and, at the end of class, was still taking notes and rushing to write down her assignments and gather her things. As a result, she tended to stuff papers into her notebooks or folded them into her books without paying close attention to where she was storing them. This led to lost assignments, and it was having a big impact on her grades. She decided to work with a coach to improve her organizational skills (coaching is described in Chapter 5). Their first step was to analyze what she was doing now. Joan was using a large three-ring binder separated by subject with an envelope at the beginning of each section. Although she tried to place worksheets, assignments, notes, etc. into the appropriate section, in her rush at the end of class she often failed to do this. Together, she and her coach designed a simpler system. They decided Joan would use two folders—one green, one red. In the green folder, she was to place all the assignments she was given for all subjects. As she finished each assignment, she immediately placed it in the red folder, ready to hand in. At the beginning of each class, Joan pulled out both folders. She looked in the red folder to see if she had any assignments to hand in for that class, and she set the green folder on her desk in preparation for any assignments she might get that period. Every day when she met with her coach, they discussed whether she remembered to follow her organizational scheme. Joan remarked that she had felt a little funny at first, with two brightly colored folders on her desk, but she felt better when a friend of hers noticed what she was doing, asked her about it, and liked the idea so much she began using the same system herself.

TABLE 4.13. Time Management

Description of skill

The capacity to estimate, allocate, and execute within time constraints.

Environmental modifications

Refer also to the suggestions under *Sustained Attention* (Table 4.9) and *Task Initiation* (Table 4.10). Time management is a higher-level executive skill that includes a number of components such as the ability to follow and make a schedule, to plan and organize, to estimate how long it takes to complete tasks, and to monitor progress in the course of completing tasks to ensure that one is "on schedule." This is a very difficult skill for many to learn because youngsters with poor time management skills tend to lack not only the ability to estimate how long it takes to do something but also lack a sense of *time urgency*—or the concept that something needs to be completed in a timely and efficient manner. These skills are needed both to ensure that students don't wait until the last minute and to ensure that they work efficiently once they begin a task. For youngsters who have weak time management skills, environmental modifications to reduce the negative effects of this weakness might include the following:

- Give youngsters a schedule to follow and prompt them at each step of the way.
- Impose time limits and provide reminders for how much time is left.
- Use cuing devices such as clocks, bells, or alarms.

Teaching the skill

There are a number of prerequisite skills youngsters need in order to manage time effectively, including the ability to tell time, the ability to make and follow a schedule, and the ability to estimate how long it takes to do something. We've already discussed making schedules under <u>Planning</u> (Table 4.11). Learning to estimate involves (1) helping the youngster understand what the task involves (e.g., the steps required to complete the task and how long it will take to do each step), and (2) a realistic sense of what the likely distracters, diversions, and roadblocks are and how they will impact the schedule and time estimates. Teaching estimation, therefore, involves having the youngster make a plan to accomplish the task and guess how long each step will take. The youngster can then compare his estimates to the actual time required. If the two numbers don't match, then some discussion should take place of the factors that contributed to the mismatch. If the youngster finds himself susceptible to distractions, then he should put in place a strategy to minimize distractions.

In terms of instilling a sense of time urgency, the easiest way to do this is by making the end point of the task a critical event or meaningful consequence. For instance, if a child is slow to get ready to go to school in the morning, if she has to walk to school if she misses the bus, then this consequence may be salient enough for her to get ready more quickly. Some parents effectively use access to fun activities to build in this sense of time urgency: for example, the budding hockey star may find it easier to get his homework done quickly if he knows that if it's not done before hockey practice, he doesn't get to go.

As with the other more complex executive skills, coaching is often an effective process for helping youngsters acquire good time management skills.

Vignette

Fred, an 11th grader, was constantly getting work done at the last minute or asking teachers to give him extensions for due dates. He had perfected the art of believable excuses—way beyond "the dog ate it" or "my computer crashed"—and he was considering writing a book on the subject that he thought would be a best-seller among his classmates. However, his teachers were losing patience with him, and he finally decided he needed to bite the bullet. One of his teachers offered to act as his coach to help him tackle the problem.

(continued)

TABLE 4.13. (*continued*)

They decided that Step 1 was for him to learn to better estimate how long it took to do things. Each day they looked at his homework for the day and Fred wrote down how long he thought it would take him to do each task. When he did his homework, he wrote down the actual start and finish time and compared reality with his estimate. Slowly Fred learned that it usually took him at least 25% longer to complete a task than he thought it would. With this knowledge, he began to improve his estimates and to plan his time better. In the process of working on this skill, he and his coach also realized that Fred had a tendency to commit himself to way too many activities. He was involved in several after-school clubs, was on the Student Council, and had a part-time job on the weekends. With his coach's help, Fred made some hard decisions about which activities he wanted to hold on to and which he should give up. This was not easy for him, but he found it did make a difference. When his dad showed up late for dinner for the fourth night in a row, Fred kidded him about how he needed to learn to "say no." His dad looked startled, and it dawned on Fred that he was learning a life skill that might help him long after he finished school.

TABLE 4.14. Goal-Directed Persistence

The capacity to have a goal, follow through to the completion of the goal, and not be put off by or distracted by competing interests.

Environmental modifications

The environmental modifications for this executive skill are similar to those for *Time Management* (Table 4.13). For youngsters with weak goal-directed persistence, accommodating this weakness means that rather than rely on them to establish a goal and persist to achieve the goal, adults both give them goals and prompt them to keep on track. For this to work effectively, the goals set should be ones that the youngsters have some motivation to work toward. Involving them as full partners in establishing those goals is often the best way to do this. If they have trouble establishing goals for themselves, giving them choices for what they might want to work toward may make this easier for them.

An effective way to enhance a youngster's motivation to work toward a goal is to make that goal as real and as visible to the youngster as possible. For instance, if parents want their son to go to college, they might arrange for him to visit likely colleges early in high school so that he has a concrete impression of the college experience that he can draw on as he continues in high school. A 16-year-old that wants to save money to buy a car might tack a picture of a car on his bedroom wall or a bulletin board by his desk.

Ideally, the goal should be in sight. With younger children, this means setting goals so that the time it takes to reach the goal is quite short. With older youngsters, ways can be found both to keep the goal in sight (like the car on the bulletin board). To help a youngster persist in his efforts to achieve a goal, giving him feedback about his progress toward the goal can help. For instance, the youngster saving for a car might keep a bar graph showing how much money he has saved so far. Revisiting the goal frequently, for example, in the course of the coaching process, can also keep the goal real for the youngster.

Teaching the skill

The most effective procedure we know of for teaching goal-directed persistence is to use a coaching process. Chapter 5 outlines this process.

Vignette

Ever since she could remember, Amy wanted to be an archeologist when she grew up. She read every book she could get her hands on. She was particularly interested in the Native American cultures of the Southwest, and she spoke quite knowledgeably on the subject to anyone who would listen. By the time she began her sophomore year in high school, however, Amy realized that the grades she was earning were probably not good enough to get her to her goal. When her parents tried to talk with her about this, she just got angry: "What does algebra have to do with archeology?" she fumed. "And why do I have to read The Red Badge of Courage? *It has nothing to do with what I'm interested in." Amy's parents, in frustration, took her to see a counselor. Once they'd established some trust between them and Amy began to value the counselor's opinion, the counselor began talking with her about her long-term goals. She persuaded her that although it seemed as though a lot of high school requirements had nothing to do with what she wanted to do when she grew up, getting poor grades would close a lot of doors for her. Amy was a smart girl, and good grades came easily to her when she was younger. She realized it would not take too much more effort for her to bring her grades up if she set that as a goal. Together, she and her counselor set some marking period goals. They talked about each subject and what grade Amy thought she could earn in that subject. They also talked about what she would have to do differently to earn those grades. Although she only saw the counselor once a week, she agreed to e-mail her counselor every day outlining her study plan. The next day, she would let her counselor know whether she had followed her plan. After about 6 weeks, she felt that she was into the routine enough so she could cut back to weekly check-ins with her counselor. By the end of the marking period, she had brought up all her grades and was close to making the honor roll. When she discussed her report card with her counselor, she set as her goal to make the honor roll by the end of the next marking period. Her parents also arranged for the family to take a vacation to Arizona. They planned to visit both some archeological sites and the campus of Arizona State University—a college with a strong archeology program that Amy wanted to check out.*

TABLE 4.15. Flexibility

Description of skill

The ability to revise plans in the face of obstacles, setbacks, new information, or mistakes. It relates to an adaptability to changing conditions.

Environmental modifications

For youngsters who tend to be inflexible, environmental modifications primarily involve reducing the demands for flexibility. These may include:

- Reducing novelty. This can be done (1) by advance familiarization with places, schedules, or activities through the use of "dry runs" or rehearsals; (2) preteaching or giving the youngster the opportunity to preview material to be presented; (3) providing advance warning, such as cuing the child in advance of transitions; (4) systematic, gradual exposure to new situations; or (5) participation in rule-based social groups to provide social experiences in a more structured setting.
- Modifying the nature of the task. This can be done by (1) decreasing the speed, volume, or complexity of information presentation; (2) breaking tasks down into component parts; (3) adapting open-ended tasks to make them more closed ended; or (4) providing the students with templates or rubrics to follow.
- Helping youngsters reframe the situation. This can be done by labeling problem situations to reduce uncertainty or creating social stories to help children understand and cope. Social stories are tailored to the individual child's unique situation and incorporate a description of the problem in a way the child identifies easily as well as a solution or coping strategy that the child can use.
- Increasing the level of support around the task. This can be done by (1) offering high frequency of reassurance or reinforcement, (2) step-by-step assistance in working through difficult problems, (3) graded exposure or guided mastery, (4) close contact at transition times, or (5) cuing the child to use coping strategies (see below).

Teaching the skill

The first step in teaching youngsters to become more flexible is to help them understand what inflexibility is and then to teach them to recognize when they feel themselves being inflexible. You might explain to a child, for instance, that being inflexible means thinking there's only one right answer or only one path to a solution when in fact there are typically several right answers or several paths. Individuals who lack flexibility tend, without even realizing it, to create an imaginary scenario of what they expect to happen and then to rehearse that scenario in their minds until it becomes a "mental set." When reality doesn't match that mental set, the outcome for those individuals is confusion, agitation, anger, or frustration. This might be analogous to how you might feel upon finding that the plane you expected to take to New York is actually going to Chicago—and you only discover this as the plane is touching down at O'Hare Airport!

- Once youngsters are able to recognize inflexibility in themselves, the next step is to teach them coping strategies for managing the emotions and the situation. Teaching coping strategies, of course, involves modeling, practice, feedback, and generalization to real settings, with cues to prompt the youngster to use the strategy until it is internalized. Coping strategies might include:
- Giving youngsters plans or rules for managing specific situations that arise frequently and cuing them to follow the plans or rules until they become internalized.
- Helping students develop "default" strategies they can fall back on.
- Providing scripts that can be used in problem situations (this could be incorporated into social stories, described above).
- Teaching relaxation strategies, thought-stopping, or attention diversion strategies (e.g., through the use of visual imagery).
- Teaching youngsters the concept of an "error factor" to reduce absolutist thinking. For instance, some children become very upset in sports situations when an umpire or referee makes a call that they think is wrong. Preparing children in advance for this by letting them know that those officiating games are "allowed" to make mistakes may reduce unhappiness when perceived bad calls are made.

(continued)

63

TABLE 4.15. *(continued)*

<u>Vignette</u>

Jeff, age 10, was a creature of habit. He struggled with transitions to new situations and always had difficulty in the first few weeks of each new grade until he became familiar with the schedule and with his teachers' expectations. In fourth grade he continued to struggle even after 2½ months. His teacher followed a schedule, but she expected increased independence on the part of her students, so they had to be more flexible in accommodating to their work production and the time they needed for help. This was very frustrating to Jeff. Each day when he came into school he expected that his teacher would do reading and language arts before recess and math right after recess. He struggled a bit with writing but looked forward to math because it was defined, black and white. When writing spilled over into math time Jeff got very upset and sometimes refused to finish. To help Jeff with this, his teacher started to check in with him every morning. If the language arts material for the day looked complex and she felt that it may run into math time, she presented an altered schedule that would help him to "reset" his expectations. She also set the criteria for his completion of language arts work, and when this was done he had the option of starting some math. Over time, she planned to work with Jeff on developing a personal schedule so that he learned to estimate how much time his work would take. The goal for Jeff was to learn that an "estimate" is just that, and hence that schedules—and Jeff—needed to have some flexibility.

TABLE 4.16. Metacognition

Description of skill

The ability to stand back and take a bird's-eye view of oneself in a situation. It is an ability to observe how you problem solve. It also includes self-monitoring and self-evaluative skills (e.g., asking yourself, "How am I doing?" or "How did I do?").

Environmental modifications

These are designed to prompt children to use analytic skills to assess how they are performing assigned tasks. They include:

- Embedding questions designed to elicit metacognition into daily classroom instruction. Here are some examples of questions teachers might ask: How did you solve that problem? Can you think of another way of doing that? What can you do to help remember that information?
- Building error monitoring into task assignments (e.g., by requiring children to show that they have checked their work when doing math computations or by having them fill out proofreading checklists before handing in writing assignments).
- Giving children assignments requiring them to use metacognitive skills. For example, they could be asked to give themselves a grade on an assignment and to explain why they feel they deserve that grade.
- Using scoring rubrics to define what a quality product or assignment will include.

Teaching the skill

Metacognition is such a broad executive skill that one specific set of procedures for teaching the skill cannot be identified. Examples of teaching procedures might include the following:

- Have children develop error-monitoring checklists and then prompt them to use them, gradually fading the prompts.
- Teach children a set of questions to ask themselves when confronted with problem situations. Here are some questions they might ask: (1) What is my problem (problem definition)? (2) What is my plan (solution strategy)? (3) Am I following my plan (self-monitoring prompt)? (4) How did I do (self-evaluation)? These questions could be written in a list form and publicly displayed. Parents or teachers could then prompt the child to go through the set of questions when problem situations arise.
- Teach the child to ask himself specific questions in problem situations, with the questions tailored to the specific problem. For instance, if a child tends to invade other children's personal space resulting in annoyance or rejection, he might be taught to ask himself, "Did I get too close?" and to move away from the other child if the answer is yes. He might also be taught that the definition of "too close" is "if the child is closer to me than two shoe lengths."
- As with many of the skills described so far, the procedure for teaching the child to use metacognitive skills includes (1) defining the skill to be learned, (2) listing the steps the child goes through in using the skill, (3) practicing the skill in a controlled setting, (4) cuing the child to use the skill in the natural environment, (5) reinforcing the child for using the skill either verbally or through the use of an incentive system, and (6) fading the cues and reinforcement.

Vignette

Sam, in second grade, made many mistakes in math. On math computation, he often failed to note the operation that he was supposed to perform; as a result he often added when he should have been subtracting or vice versa. His teacher kept handing papers back with low grades and reminders to "Watch the signs!" When his performance did not improve, she decided that he needed to learn a procedure that would help him do the problems correctly. She taught him to say to himself as he began each problem, "Am I adding or subtracting?" She and Sam practiced this a lot; she also sent a note home to his parents so that they could use the same process to help him with his homework. With enough practice, he began making a lot fewer mistakes.

(continued)

TABLE 4.16. *(continued)*

Joe, in fifth grade, also tended to make careless mistakes in math, but his problem was different. When he had to solve multistep problems, he stopped after the first step and gave that number as his answer. His teacher also taught him a procedure. Now, when he has to solve a math problem, he first figures out each step and then writes down a notation for that step as a reminder. For instance, he's given the problem, "If you buy 5 candy bars for 60 cents each, how much change should you get back from 5 dollars?" His teacher taught him to say, "First I multiple 5 times 60 cents," then write down an M for multiply on his paper. Then he says, "I take that number and subtract it from 5 dollars," writing an S for subtraction on the paper. As he completes each step, he crosses out the letter describing that step.

5

Coaching Students
with Executive Skill Deficits

In the previous chapter, we described several general intervention strategies for enhancing executive skills or minimizing the negative effect of weak executive skills, as well as specific interventions targeted to individual executive skill deficits. Through our work with children and adults who had traumatic brain injuries we were well aware of the relationship between frontal lobe injuries and deficits in executive skills even in so-called minor head injuries. We also recognized executive skill weaknesses in many of the children with attention disorders with whom we worked.

Coaching grew out of an intervention that we originally described as mentoring. We recommended this strategy for some of the attention-deficit/hyperactivity disorder (ADHD) and learning disabled students whom we saw that needed help with organizing and remembering their materials and structuring their time. Hallowell and Ratey (1994), in their book *Driven to Distraction*, briefly described a coach as an "individual standing on the sideline with a whistle around his or her neck barking out encouragement, directions, and reminders to the player in the game. . . . Mainly, the coach keeps the player focused on the task at hand and offers encouragement along the way"(p. 226). We liked this notion of a coach and felt that it fit well with our idea of mentoring. At around the same time Russell A. Barkley (1993) presented an outline of his theory on the relationship between executive skills weaknesses and ADHD. A third element contributing to our coaching model emerged from the behavioral literature on correspondence training. Defined by Paniagua (1992) as a chain of behaviors that "include a verbalization or report about past or future behavior and the corresponding nonverbal behavior," one aspect of correspondence training involves making a verbal commitment to engage in a behavior at some later point. This verbal commitment increases the likelihood that the behavior will actually take place.

By weaving these various elements together into a system we felt that the coaching process could be an effective intervention for students. We developed each stage of the coaching model to correspond to an aspect of executive skills and incorporated the strategy of correspondence training by including in each coaching session a verbal and written commitment on the part of the student to carry out the objectives for that day. Thus, coaching was developed as a systematic training process that initially provides a person with access to the executive skills that he or she needs to accomplish a goal. The process serves, via the coach and the associated documentation, as a "lend-lease frontal lobe," available on a temporary basis as the student develops his or her executive skills.

The coaching process embodies some unique aspects. To succeed, the process requires the student's willing and active participation at each step, a factor not always in evidence in intervention strategies with children. Related to this, coaching is continuously collaborative, encouraging the child or adolescent to make decisions and choices. The process is designed to be managed by the student and the coach, independent of parental supervision. This can serve to diffuse conflict or criticism that may have developed around performance issues.

As an intervention, coaching operates simultaneously at three levels. The first level involves the accomplishment of a task or set of tasks satisfying some performance standard in the student's environment (e.g., parent or teacher expectations; grades). The second level continuously draws a relationship between day-to-day (or minute-to-minute) tasks and the student's longer-term goal, satisfying his or her own sense of accomplishment and efficacy. The third level teaches, on a daily basis, a set of executive skills and over time gradually fades the coach's role and increases the student's active use of these skills. In addition, the coach encourages the development of new goals and the student's use of executive skills to achieve these goals, thus promoting generalization and transfer.

Given the active and collaborative nature of the approach, coaching is most successful with students who are willing and active participants and who have made a commitment to change. Hence, when reluctant students have been "talked into" or worse yet coerced into participation in the coaching process, it is unlikely to succeed. We have found that when younger students are approached with a problem that the adult has noted ("Caitlin, it seems that completion of your math work in class is a problem. Would you be willing to work with me on a plan to complete your work?"), they usually are willing to participate in the coaching process. When individual coaching is the intervention of choice with late middle school and high school students, the choice of participation and who will be the coach rests largely with them.

In this chapter we describe coaching—a process that we believe has broad applications to students of different ages with a variety of executive skill deficits. Coaching was originally conceptualized as an intervention strategy for teenagers with attention disorders (Dawson & Guare, 1998); we also believe it can be a highly successful intervention for students with executive skill weaknesses, whether or not they have attention disorders. For a more complete discussion of the process, as well as the forms designed to accompany the process, please see our original publication, *Coaching the ADHD Student* (Dawson & Guare, 1998).

Coaching is a process in which an adult works with students to set important school-related goals and then to ensure that the students' actions and behaviors on a daily basis are consistent with those goals and, in fact, bring them closer to achieving them. Coaching with children of all ages is a two-step process. In Step 1, the student selects a goal or a set of goals he or she wants to work on. In Step 2, the student identifies tasks he or she needs to do on a daily basis in order to achieve that goal. This coaching process is summarized in Table 5.1 and is also described in more detail below.

STEP 1: CONDUCT A GOAL-SETTING SESSION

The first step in coaching is to help the student identify a goal she would like to work on. The goal selected will depend in part on the age and developmental level of the child, in part on the child's interests, and in part on what parents or teachers think are important behaviors for the youngster to work on.

With elementary-age children, the goal will generally be something that can be accomplished on a daily basis. For instance, one student may decide he wants to work on getting daily assignments completed on time. Another student may decide she wants to work on raising her hand before speaking in class.

By the middle school level, some students are ready to set somewhat longer-term goals. We often recommend that students at this age set marking period goals. For instance, an eighth grader may decide she wants to work toward earning a B in science, her most difficult subject. Or a seventh-grade boy for whom discipline is an issue may decide he wants to finish the marking period having earned no more than three after-school detentions for talking back to his teacher.

TABLE 5.1. Overview of the Coaching Process

Step 1. Conduct a goal-setting session.

This session should include three components:

- Setting a goal. This may be a daily, weekly, or marking-period goal, depending on the age and developmental level of the student. Older high school students should be encouraged to set a long-term goal that addresses their plans following high school completion.
- Identifying potential obstacles to achieving the goal and ways to overcome the obstacles.
- Writing a plan for achieving the goal.

Step 2. Hold daily coaching sessions.

The purpose of the daily coaching session is to make a plan for the day. There is some flexibility in how daily coaching sessions are conducted, but in general, the first part of the session is spent reviewing the previous day's plan and the second part is spent designing the plan for the current day. This may include asking the student the following questions:

- Did you complete the tasks you said you were going to do yesterday?
- Were you satisfied with the amount of time and effort you put in to those tasks?
- What do you have to do for today? (Make a list.)
- When are you going to do each of the tasks you have identified?
- Are there other activities or responsibilities you have to work around in order to complete today's plan?
- Are there long-term projects or exams coming up that we need to begin planning for?
- Given how things are going, are you on target to achieve the goal you set in Step 1?

At the high school level, we still recommend that students set marking period goals, but many students are also ready to begin thinking more long term. For example, the coach may help them establish a goal related to what they want to do after high school.

The developmental differences in coaching involve not only how long term the goals may be but also whether the process is chosen by the adult or by the student. Whereas in high school we believe it works best as a student choice, at the elementary and middle school level coaching can be integrated into the student's daily schedule (e.g., during time in the resource room or a study hall). In all cases, we recommend that the coach be some-one the student enjoys working with—whenever possible we recommend that students themselves identify whom they want to work with as a coach.

Once the goal is established, this first phase of the coaching process includes a discussion of the potential obstacles that students may encounter in their efforts to reach their goal as well as the steps they may need to follow in order to achieve the goals. Coaches may be able to help students identify supports both within the school and at home they can draw on to help them reach their goals. For instance, if an elementary student is working on completing work in a timely fashion, she may arrange to do some of her seatwork in a quiet corner of the classroom or in the resource room in order to minimize distractions. At the middle school level, students may decide to stay after school and participate in an after-school homework club if they have set as a goal getting homework handed in on time and completed. For high school students who may identify earning certain grades in specific subjects, coaches should discuss with them what grades they earned in the past and what they think they need to do differently in order to reach their goals.

While this discussion takes place at the beginning of the coaching process, the goal set is frequently referred back to as coaching gets under way. This is particularly important if the executive skill being worked on relates to "goal-directed persistence," since it's very important to keep the long-term goal clearly in mind (or in working memory) as the process unfolds.

STEP 2: HOLD DAILY COACHING SESSIONS

Once a coaching relationship has been established and a goal set, students and coaches meet on a daily basis to make plans for what they will work on that day to bring them closer to their goal and to assess how successful their efforts have been. Generally, this is done by the coach asking the student a series of questions designed to help him formulate a plan for the day. When the coaching process is underway, the first part of the session involves reviewing the plan made the day before and evaluating the student's success at following the plan. Then a new plan is drawn up. In so doing, the coach helps the student think about the plan in depth, both to identify all the necessary steps as well as to anticipate what problems the student may encounter in following the plan.

For many daily plans, there are two key ingredients that students need to include. First, they need to specify exactly *what* they are going to do. Secondly, they need to specify *when* they are going to do each task. There is a body of research (e.g., Paniagua, 1992) that demonstrates that making a public commitment to perform a task vastly increases the likelihood that the individual making the commitment will actually carry out the task. *Correspondence* involves the agreement between a verbal description of what one will do and actually doing it, that is, between what I say and what I do. One aspect of correspondence training involves a verbal statement that one will engage in a behavior at some later point. This verbal commitment, particularly if public, increases the likelihood that the behavior will actually take place.

The specific plan the coach and student draw up, of course, depends on the goal being worked on. Again, with younger children, since goals tend to be quite simple and precise, the plan may be easy to formulate and quite straightforward. For instance, if the goal of an elementary-age child is to remember to bring home at the end of the day the materials needed for homework, then the coach and student together might make a list of what those materials are and the child can agree to check off the list as he gathers the appropriate materials to put in his backpack at the end of the day. For this particular example, holding the coaching session at the end of the day will make it easier for the coach and child to make their plan and for the child to follow through on it.

With older students, since the goals tend to be longer term and more complex, the plan is likely to be somewhat more complicated. For instance, with high school students who are trying to develop good planning/organization or time management skills, developing the plan may include reviewing with the student the assignments that are due the next day as well as any upcoming tests or long-term projects or papers the student needs to be working on. Part of the planning process might include breaking down long-term assignments into subtasks and assigning due dates to each subtask, as well as determining what needs to get done by the next day. Then the student makes a list of everything she needs to do before tomorrow and identifies when each task will be done. It may be the job of the coach to push the student to be as specific as possible, both in terms of what the student will do and when she will do it. For instance, if the student says she will study for her science test right after supper, the coach may want to pin the student down both in terms of how much time she plans to spend studying but also *how* she intends to study (e.g., by making flash cards of key terms, writing out questions on index cards with answers on the back, going back and highlighting notes, or creating a graphic to visually organize notes). This degree of specificity will be more essential with some students than others.

While it is the job of a coach to help students plan, problem solve, and evaluate their efforts, it is also the job of the coach to act as a mentor and cheerleader. For some students, having an adult cheering them on as they reach toward goals that seem lofty to them can make the difference between success and failure. Coaches can also act as go-betweens or mediators when students encounter problems related to the coaching goals.

The applications of coaching are many and varied, but to give the reader a sense of how the process works, let's create a dialogue that might take place between Joe, a high school student, and his coach. Let's assume the following conversation takes place in the first daily coaching session.

COACH: Joe, you've set as a goal for the marking period to bring your English grade up to a B. This will take some work on your part, since last marking period you got a C. Do you remember what you said you were going to try to do differently to improve your grade?

JOE: Yes, I'm going to study for my weekly vocabulary tests, I'm going to stay on top of my reading assignments, and I'm not going to leave papers until the night before they're due so I'll have time to edit and revise.

COACH: Excellent. All good ideas. If you can follow through on them, I'm sure your grade will improve. The coaching we're going to do should help you do this. What we will do when we get together every day is to make a plan for the day that will help you reach your goal. So why don't we begin by taking a look at what's coming up in English. Do you have anything due for that class tomorrow?

JOE: Yes, I'm supposed to read the first chapter of *Lord of the Flies*.

COACH: Anything else—any study questions to answer or reader response you have to write?

JOE: No, except we're supposed to keep an eye out for something that might *foreshadow* later events in the book.

COACH: How are you planning on doing that?

JOE: Well, Ms. Hancock told us we should look for tensions between characters that might be likely to get worse as the book goes along. Or maybe look for things that are important to characters or maybe personality traits or character flaws that might get them in trouble . . . things like that.

COACH: Sounds good. How are you going to keep track of your ideas?

JOE: I have my own paperback copy of the book, so I thought I would put the letter F in the margin by each detail that might be foreshadowing.

COACH: Sounds like a good plan. When do you think you'll be able to do this assignment?

JOE: I was planning on doing it in my seventh-period study hall.

COACH: Do you think that will give you enough time?

JOE: I think so, but if not, I can finish it after basketball practice and just before dinner.

COACH: Okay. Let's talk about upcoming English assignments. What's on the horizon?

JOE: (*consulting his agenda book*) I have a vocabulary test on Thursday, and by next Monday I have to have read the first three chapters of *Lord of the Flies* and write a reader response.

COACH: So you have three nights before the vocabulary test. Have you thought about how you might use the time to study?

JOE: (*a little sheepishly*) I wasn't even going to think about this until Wednesday night. That's a big improvement over last marking period, when I didn't study at all!

COACH: There's actually some good research to show that spreading out studying into several short sessions is a more effective way to learn material than to cram the night before. But tell you what, let's use this week as a baseline. Why don't you plan to study the night before and we'll look at your quiz grade. Then we can decide if you might want to try a different approach next week. . . . So, what's your plan with reading the rest of *Lord of the Flies* and writing the response?

JOE: I thought I'd read the other two chapters on Saturday and write the response on Sunday night.

COACH: Let me make a suggestion. You may want to look at how many pages you'll have to read for the second and third chapters and divide the total by the number of days you have left until Sunday. If you can read a little each day, it'll be easier to stay on top of the reading. Maybe you can take advantage of little pieces of time, say, in study hall or while you're waiting for dinner.

JOE: I like that idea. I'm a slow reader so what's gotten me in trouble before is not allowing enough time to do all the reading *and* write the response.

COACH: You've left the paper until the night before it's due. One of your strategies was not to do that.

JOE: Oh, I meant leaving *big* papers until the last minute. This is just a little thing I should be able to whip off in less than an hour.

COACH: Do you need help thinking about how to write your paper?

JOE: Nah, I'm good at that. I did lousy before because I'd only do half the reading and then I'd try to fake it. If I can get the reading done, the paper should be a piece of cake.

COACH: All right. I think we have a plan for today. With the work you have set for English, do you think you'll be able to fit in your other homework, too?

JOE: I think so. English has always been bad because I don't like it and I kept putting it off. If this'll help me stay on top of the work, I should be fine.

COACH: Great! I think this process will work well for you. You're off to a good start. Writing down assignments and keeping track of what's due when is an important part of the process, and it seems like you do that well.

JOE: Yeah. Well, having enough teachers drum into me the importance of writing things down finally got through to me. See you tomorrow, "Coach"!

The next session might begin by having the coach and Joe pull out the plan they created the day before and review it to see if Joe followed the plan—both in terms of doing what he said he was going to do and in terms of the time commitment. If Joe deviates from the plan, then the coach would be wise to explore with Joe what got in the way and to keep those obstacles in mind when making future plans. Then a new plan is drawn up. The coach should again review with Joe both immediate assignments and the long-term assignments he also needs to stay on top of. Each day the coach should ask Joe if he's been assigned anything long term that he needs to be thinking about. And even though Joe's goal only pertains to bringing up his English grade, it will be important for Joe not to lose sight of the work he has to do for other classes, as well as other obligations such as basketball games, any job he may have, or any family obligations that will take time away from studying and reaching his goal.

Initially, coaching sessions should occur daily. As can be seen from the above scenario, it does not need to be a long process and can fairly quickly become a routine. Consistency is critical, however, both for the student and the coach. Over time, daily coaching sessions can be gradually faded, first by having the student and coach meet every other day, perhaps, and eventually reducing the sessions to once every week or every other week. If the fading procedure leads to the student's failure to stay on track, then sessions need to be scheduled more frequently again.

The most effective coaching we have seen takes place in the school with an adult the youngster knows well and is comfortable with acting as the student's coach. We have known students who have selected other students to act as their coaches, but when this is done, we recommend that an adult serve as "backup coach" to monitor the process and step in when problems arise.

We also think the process has group applications. Many middle schools and high schools assign students to "advisor groups" that meet daily or frequently (e.g., during homeroom period). With some modifications, including group instruction in how the coaching process works and a training period to get the process up and running, we think group coaching can be successful, either by pairing students in a peer coaching model or having the teacher lead the group in setting individual goals and reporting back to the group students' success in meeting those goals. Group applications, of course, have the added advantage of enabling the classroom teacher to address the needs of many students without having to allot individual time to each one.

BUILDING COACHING INTO THE STUDENT'S EDUCATIONAL PROGRAM

We see coaching as having a number of applications in the school setting. For students of almost any age struggling with independent work management, effective use of time, or self-regulation of behavior, coaching may play a role, and we have seen it used effectively as a component of Individualized Education Plans (IEPs) and 504 plans. In terms of establishing a coaching intervention in school there are a number of considerations:

• Does the problem to be solved lend itself to a coaching intervention? A reading problem would not lend itself to coaching, but in most cases an executive problem would.

• Is the student a willing and active participant? With all students, but particularly those in middle and high school, the viability of coaching depends on the student's active choice to be involved.

• Can a good fit between student and coach be achieved? With older students, we ask them to select their coach from among school staff. Younger children are more open to suggestions, but they must indicate comfort with the person who will be their coach.

• Does the prospective coach understand the commitment? Once the process has begun, the actual daily contact ranges from 5 to 10 minutes. Despite this seemingly brief encounter, consistency is key; if the coach becomes haphazard in his or her commitment, the intervention rapidly fails. Similarly, if the student's immediate success is taken as a sign that the problem has resolved and coaching can be discontinued, the problem frequently resurfaces.

• Is there a plan for gradually fading the intervention along with continuing measurement of the target behavior to ensure that the student has acquired the skill and can manage independently? When coaching is chosen as an intervention, we recommend that a written plan including the participants, goals chosen, type and frequency of contact, and recording format be developed and that a brief summary of the results be included. Such a record is an important component of an IEP or a 504 plan and can help to determine if this is a viable intervention strategy.

6

Classroom-Wide Interventions

Up until now, we have discussed interventions to address executive skill deficits solely in terms of individual students with executive skill impairments. However, as any teacher or educator can attest, in any classroom numerous children will exhibit difficulties associated with executive functioning. To meet the needs of all these children on an individual basis becomes time consuming and labor intensive. In fact, the most frequent question raised by teachers when we talk with them about designing interventions to address weak executive skills is "But where will I find the time?"

We believe the process of helping youngsters develop more effective executive skills can be streamlined by putting in place classroom-wide procedures and interventions that will have the effect of addressing multiple problems in many children simultaneously. Not only will this save time for teachers, it will also reduce demands on teachers' own executive skills, particularly working memory (e.g., remembering to cue individual students to follow their own personal program of executive skill development). A variety of strategies that have classroom-wide implications are addressed below.

CLASSROOM ROUTINES

One way to incorporate executive skill development in the classroom is through the use of daily routines designed either to reduce demands on executive skills or to teach students to use their executive skills more effectively. Routines most often instituted by teachers include the following:

- Beginning-of-the-day routines to accomplish tasks such as (1) handing in homework, (2) getting work materials ready for the day, or (3) making a plan or schedule for tasks to be accomplished. Some teachers we know, for instance, have their students immediately get out their homework and place it on their desks when they arrive in class for the day or for the period (in the case of middle school and high school settings). They then either collect the homework or walk around the room with their rank books making a notation for homework completion for each student.

- End-of-the-day routines to accomplish tasks such as (1) making sure homework assignments are written in daily planners or agenda books, (2) making sure students have all the materials they need to take home with them, (3) reviewing instructions for assignments or reminding students of things they need to remember to do for the following day, or (4) tidying up work spaces so that the next day can begin smoothly. Some teachers find this can be accomplished most efficiently by pairing students and having them check on each other.

Teachers who incorporate these kinds of routines in their classroom begin each school year by teaching the routines in a systematic fashion. Initially this process may seem time consuming and may appear to take time away from content instruction, but once the routines become automatic they are, in fact, time-saving devices. Teachers we have talked to who use such routines estimate that they take no more than 5 minutes at the beginning and end of the school day. When the routines are initially introduced, they should be accompanied by a checklist or cuing sheet for each student. After the process has been introduced by the teacher and practiced regularly for a while (e.g., 1–2 months), the teacher can begin cuing students to use their checklists to follow the routine. It will be necessary for the teacher to periodically evaluate effectiveness either by directly monitoring relevant behaviors (e.g., on-time homework; assignments in agenda) or by pairing students to coach/monitor each other.

CLASSROOM RULES

All teachers have a set of rules by which they run their classrooms. The most effective teachers make these rules explicit so that students fully understand the protocols for classroom behavior and performance expectations. Teachers can establish class rules that help students develop executive skills, particularly those related to behavior regulation such as inhibition of impulses and self-regulation of affect. As with classroom routines, teachers teach the rules explicitly in the beginning of the year and have students practice them. Table 6.1 provides an example of a teaching procedure.

TABLE 6.1. A Procedure for Teaching Class Rules

1. Tell the class the rule. ("The rule in this class is: Raise your hand and wait for the teacher to call on you.")
2. Practice the rule. ("I'm going to ask some questions so that we can practice the hand raising.")
3. This can be turned into a game by using positive reinforcement (e.g., by tossing students pieces of candy for following the rule successfully).
4. Cue the class to follow the rule. ("Okay, class, remember our rule about raising hands before speaking.")
5. Fade the cue. ("What's the rule?")

Many teachers use daily or weekly class meetings to discuss issues and concerns that come up over the course of the school year. This process, too, can incorporate executive skill development. Using this process, teachers can solicit assistance from the class in terms of defining problem behaviors and designing solutions, thereby encouraging the development of executive skills both in identifying problems and solving them. The teacher might begin a class meeting by saying, for instance, "I've noticed we've been having a lot of trouble with students saying things without thinking to other students in a way that hurts their feelings. What do you think we could do about this?" This same process, by the way, can be used to enlist students' assistance in designing effective classroom routines (e.g., "A lot of students have been forgetting to hand in their homework on time. Do you think we could develop a procedure to make it easier for students to remember to hand in assignments?").

ORGANIZATIONAL SYSTEMS

Many teachers develop uniform systems to help students keep their work organized. This might include establishing procedures for writing down assignments, completing long-term projects or reports, keeping notebooks organized, or developing a folder system or color codes to help students keep track of finished and unfinished homework and/or class assignments. It may also include organizing the physical space of the classroom to make it easier to keep track of materials or manage time. Some teachers keep separate bins in their classrooms where students are expected to hand in specific assignments. Teachers may also reserve the same spot on the blackboard for listing homework assignments or other reminders they want students to be aware of. By giving students organizational systems, teachers help them learn the benefits of having orderly processes for keeping track of materials and keeping work spaces neat. Teachers may want to discuss with students the ways they organize their materials and work spaces at home, perhaps having them draw pictures to depict how they organize their bedrooms or study areas.

While teachers, particularly at a middle school level, typically have some sort of organizational system for students to follow, these systems often vary from teacher to teacher and there may be some reluctance to give up one's own system in favor of another's. For students, this may mean adapting to a number of organizational schemes, at a time when learning and internalizing even one scheme may be a challenge. One option chosen by some schools is to adopt a grade-wide or school-wide system for all students to ensure that they acquire at least a basic set of skills.

INTEGRATING EXECUTIVE SKILL DEVELOPMENT INTO DAILY INSTRUCTION

Once teachers become aware of the importance of executive skills in the long-term success of students, they will find ways to integrate this knowledge into daily teaching. This is most easily done by asking questions that encourage students to think about how they think, learn, and plan. Examples of such questions follow:

- "How are you going to remember to ask your mother to sign your permission form?"
- "What can you do to remind yourself to raise your hand before talking?"
- "This is a big assignment. Why don't you write down the steps you need to follow to finish it."
- "What can you do to help yourself keep working until the job's done?"
- "If you don't understand an assignment, what are some things you can do to figure out what to do?"
- "You made a lot of spelling mistakes on the last book report you handed in. What can you do to reduce these mistakes in the next report?"
- "How long do you think it will take to finish this? Let's see if you're right."

If students have difficulty generating solutions, teachers can provide a few suggestions to start the process. Students will also find it helpful if their solutions are recorded for future reference. Before a triggering event (e.g., sending permission slips home) strategies can be reviewed and effectiveness monitored by return of permission slips. Some of this skill instruction, for example, time estimation, can be built into the teaching process on a regular basis. Thus, prior to independent work in class the teacher could regularly have students estimate completion time and reinforce students for accurate estimation.

Teachers who "think aloud" when confronted with problems to be solved are engaged in modeling the use of executive skills. Math teachers have become particularly adept at this, since this has become acknowledged as a "best practice" in math instruction. But the same process can be used with other tasks to which students are assigned (e.g., grammar exercises, how to select topics for projects, or science experiments). When students get stuck and ask their teacher for assistance, he or she may say, "Let me show you how I might think my way through that problem," and then proceed to talk his or her way through the task to model that kind of metacognitive thinking.

Especially as students approach middle school, we often expect them to employ on their own executive skills they may not have learned. These include strategies for studying for tests or completing long-term projects, as well as the organizational skills required to complete longer writing assignments. We believe these skills all need to be taught explicitly. Thus, when long-term assignments are introduced, the projects should be broken down into subtasks, with task requirements and due dates attached to each subtask. Over time, students can be asked to assume more and more of the planning process themselves, but this process needs to be supervised to ensure that youngsters truly are acquiring the skills and not relying on parents or not simply waiting until the last minute and then "pulling an all-nighter." The process also needs to be contained in a rubric that will serve as an additional cue and checklist.

We know of very few students who have been explicitly taught how to study for tests. Students with high-functioning executive skills often design their own study strategies, but most students we know have no study strategies other than rereading the text or "going over class notes." We recommend that teachers take time during class to teach students how to study for tests. This should be done in the context of real class exams and not simply as a study skills exercise. Furthermore, test results should be analyzed with students so that they understand what worked or didn't work in their study process and so that improvements can be made as the school year goes along. Having students systematically try different study methods, both individual and group, can help them identify the strategies that work most effectively for them.

Teachers who use cooperative learning as an instructional method can also incorporate executive skill development into this process. Cooperative learning groups offer at least two different means for intervention. At the level of environmental modification/accommodation, group composition can be determined based on the particular executive skills of certain students. For example, it may be helpful to place a student who has difficulty with project completion in a group with a good planner and with a student who has goal-directed persistence. In addition, depending on the resources provided by the teacher to the group (e.g., rubrics and templates), the stronger members of the group may be able to mentor or coach the weaker student through parts of the process. This can be done by designating specific tasks, providing cues and support along the way, and modeling. Teachers could also address executive skill development more directly by establishing cooperative groups for the purpose of learning or fine tuning a set of executive skills (e.g., the types of skills needed to take a project from start-up through finished product). While project completion would be one outcome of the cooperative learning activity, an equally important outcome would be the acquisition of the executive skills necessary to complete the project successfully.

VARIATIONS ON COACHING

As described in Chapter 5, coaching, while not requiring a great deal of time, is nonetheless a fairly labor-intensive process since it involves a one-on-one interaction between a student and an adult coach. Several variations lend themselves to class-wide application.

Goal Setting

Some teachers have students set marking period goals and then check in with them on a weekly basis to determine how they are progressing toward those goals. Goals may be academic (e.g., earning a B in a subject for the marking period) or behavioral (e.g., not getting in trouble for talking with friends in class).

Group Coaching

Middle schools that employ homerooms or advisor programs where teachers have opportunities to interact with students outside of content area classes can employ a group coaching process during those sessions. This could involve having the teacher go around the group quickly, asking each student to report on what his or her work plan for the day or homework is or how well he or she followed the plan from the previous day. Or the teacher might establish a group goal that everyone is working on and have each student report progress toward that goal. Some middle schools don't use this approach with all students but may place identified at-risk students in advisor or homeroom groups where coaching can be employed to build study habits and time management skills. Coaching can also be built into before or after school "homework clubs." Some schools that employ homework clubs make them purely voluntary, whereas others require the participation of students earning low grades or consistently failing to hand in homework.

Reciprocal Coaching

This involves teaching students how to coach each other and then pairing them together for daily coaching sessions. In this model, each student acts as a coach for his or her partner. This is another way to structure homeroom or advisor groups. A variation on this is a cross-age model in which older students who have executive skill weaknesses themselves are taught to act as mentors for younger students and, through this process, build on their own executive skills.

With respect to reciprocal coaching, we need to make a distinction between peer coaching and peer tutoring. A process in which one student coaches another may appear similar to peer tutoring in that one student works with another to help develop a skill. However, in peer coaching the emphasis is on process rather than product. The goal is not mastery of an academic skill but mastery of the executive skills needed for a student to become an effective, independent learner. In reciprocal coaching the roles are roughly equal and the students learn both by having a coach who monitors their application of executive skills and by applying these same criteria with their peer so that the process is continually reinforced. In the peer coaching model, reciprocity is not a key element. Rather, the peer coach is a mentor and functions in a manner similar to an adult coach. Although the primary objective is not enhanced skill development for the coach, this is likely to be a by-product.

CAVEATS

A review of this chapter by teachers may produce the comment that they've attempted to use procedures such as the ones described but have not found them to be effective. In our experience, in order for class-wide procedures to be implemented successfully, the following things must happen:

- The process must be taught explicitly, with lots of opportunity to practice the procedure. Teachers may say, "I told them how to study for the test, but they didn't do what I suggested." Students must be walked through the process, and they must be given performance feedback so they know how well they are learning the process and how they need to improve.
- The process or procedure must be monitored daily for far longer than many teachers believe is necessary. If the process involves, for instance, getting students to write

down assignments in agenda books, we have found that teachers need to have a system to allow for daily checks, for example, students checking each other. The checks can be gradually faded, but some students will need those daily checks for longer than others and teachers need to be aware of and responsive to individual differences.

• The process must be designed, described, and taught carefully and with attention to detail. Otherwise, this will leave some students confused while for others it will create loopholes that will enable them to "beat the system."

• If the system fails, teachers should redesign the system. A teacher may say, "The rest of the class is able to follow this procedure. Lisa must just not want to do it." Motivation may be an element of an individual student's inability to perform a task or skill, but we have found that this problem is best addressed through a carefully designed system, with additional controls introduced for those students who don't respond well to the "looser" systems that may work for a majority of the class.

This chapter is only a brief introduction to the ways class-wide interventions can be designed to foster executive skills. Experienced classroom teachers will be able to envision variations on these suggestions that can be tailored to fit their own teaching style or the needs of the students they teach.

7

Applications to Specific Populations

Barring some catastrophic event, children are born with the capacity to develop executive skills. The extent to which they develop these skills depends on genetic and environmental factors, and each child falls along a continuum with regard to executive skills. Hence, children will have strengths and weaknesses. They may be very poor at sustaining attention or initiating tasks, or they can have mild problems, or they can be very good at these skills. In some cases, their weaknesses will be sufficient to interfere with daily living and school demands. Parents and teachers need to recognize the severity of the problem in the children they work with and adjust their efforts accordingly.

Children with executive skill weaknesses fall into at least three categories. We have suggested that these weaknesses can occur in the absence of any currently recognized disorder or "diagnosis." Thus, one category comprises those children who simply have weaknesses in one or more executive skills in the absence of any other condition or disorder. A second category comprises those children who, by virtue of a certain condition or diagnosis, are likely to have a number of executive skill deficits. This category includes children with acquired brain injuries, some autism spectrum disorders, and ADHD. The third category includes children whose suspected executive skill weaknesses are confounded by other complex learning and/or social-emotional factors. We consider these categories in turn in the following sections.

EXECUTIVE SKILL WEAKNESSES IN THE ABSENCE OF A RECOGNIZED DISORDER

With respect to the first category, we have found it useful to think of strengths and weaknesses in children (and adults) as a normal and expected condition. In some cases, the weaknesses will be minor and compensated for by the child's strengths. In other cases, the skill deficit will be sufficient to interfere with some aspect of work or problem solving. It is important for parents and teachers to be aware of the strengths and weaknesses of their children in order to accurately tailor their own support only to those areas where support is needed. It is also important for adults to be aware of their own strengths and weaknesses. We have worked with children whose relative weakness in an executive skill was made to seem much more extreme by virtue of a parent's or teacher's strong skill in the same area. For example, a highly organized teacher may find mild disorganization in a child more problematic than a teacher who does not value organization as highly.

DISORDERS THAT IMPACT EXECUTIVE FUNCTIONING

Acquired Brain Injury

Acquired brain injury involves an impairment of brain functioning as a result of either an external event such as head trauma or an internal event such as a stroke, oxygen deprivation, or infection. As Savage and Wolcott (1994) and Ylvisaker, Szerkeres, and Hartwick (1994) indicate, deficits in executive functions are frequently a central feature of acquired brain injury. Even in cases where other functions have been spared, weaknesses in executive skills can have a major impact on the child's performance and can present a significant impediment to independent functioning. Effects are not limited to the most severe injuries. Children with so-called mild brain injuries (e.g., those resulting from concussions) also demonstrate problems with executive skills (Frey, 1994). In addition, for children who may have acquired their injury early in life and who are being evaluated at relatively young ages, it is important not to assume that absence of evidence is evidence of absence. Demands on executive skills are limited in early childhood. Deficits may be revealed only as the child ages and demands come "on line."

Autism Spectrum Disorders

Executive skill deficits also have been identified in Asperger syndrome (AS) and more broadly in the autism spectrum disorders, particularly high-functioning autism (HFA) (Ozonoff & Griffith, 2000). Work in this area is only in the preliminary stages, and there is no specific pattern of executive skill weaknesses identified with AS or HFA or evidence that the disorders can be distinguished on the basis of particular executive skill patterns. In our clinical experience, children with AS and with nonverbal learning disabilities (NLD) often demonstrate problems with self-regulation of affect, metacognition, and flexibility. That the AS and NLD groups might share characteristics is not surprising in light of research suggesting broad similarities between the two groups (Rourke & Tsatsanis, 2000).

Attention-Deficit/Hyperactivity Disorder

If executive skill deficits are prevalent in acquired brain injury, autism spectrum disorders, and nonverbal learning disabilities, they are central in ADHD. Barkley (1997), in our opinion, makes a compelling case that goal-directed persistence is deficient in the individual with ADHD. The source of this problem is a weakness in self-regulation and the executive skills that form the basis for this ability. Thus, in the Barkley model, ADHD is fundamentally a deficit in executive skills. However, even if one does not subscribe specifically to Barkley's theory, there is a general consensus in the literature on ADHD that executive skills play a central role in the disorder. Considering the number of children who have the disorder (conservatively estimated at 3–5%), the result is a significant population with executive skill deficits.

Sleep Disorders and Sleep Deprivation

For children who fall into this second category, where executive skill weaknesses are associated with certain conditions, it is important to be cognizant of this relationship. When a child presents with one of these conditions a thorough assessment of executive skills should be completed. When deficits are identified intervention plans should address both current and future needs since these deficits, with the exception of sleep deprivation, remain part of a condition that is not likely to simply resolve over time. In addition, children with these conditions are at risk for other academic problems that may be aggravated by executive skill deficits.

The impact of sleep on school performance has only recently come to the attention of educators (Wahlstrom, 1999). Educational policy makers have become increasingly aware of the changing sleep patterns found in normal adolescents and the implications this has for school start time. A survey by the National Sleep Foundation (1999) conducted with parents found that 60% of children under the age of 18 complain of daytime sleepiness and 15% report falling asleep in class. More than 7% of youngsters between the ages of 12 and 19 report symptoms associated with delayed sleep onset syndrome, a circadian rhythm disorder that results in difficulty falling asleep at normal bedtime hours (Pelayo, Thorpy, & Glovinsky, 1988). All of this suggests that a significant portion of school-age children are going to school sleep deprived. The impact of sleep deprivation on executive functioning is direct, since the prefrontal cortex helps regulate sleep, arousal, and attention. Youngsters who are sleep deprived have been shown to have difficulty initiating and persisting at tasks, especially those viewed as tedious or "boring." They also have difficulty with complex tasks that require planning or goal-directed persistence, particularly when the goals are abstract and the rewards are delayed (Dahl, 1999). All of these, of course, are executive skills. Assessing the presence of sleep problems when presented with a child with executive skill problems is essential: the remedy may be ensuring more adaptive sleep patterns rather than putting in place interventions directly related to executive functioning.

COMPLICATED CASES

The third category comprises children who present with complicated issues of which executive skills may be one aspect. These cases manifest in at least two ways. Some children are initially referred for evaluation of executive skills with the presumption that weaknesses in such skills are at the heart of a problem, for example, that weaknesses in task initiation or goal-directed persistence result in poor work production. We recently saw a young woman with work production problems whose ratings on executive skills checklists by parents and teachers were well within the clinical range. A classroom observation confirmed problems with organization, task initiation, and goal-directed persistence. Observation also revealed little peer interaction and apparent disinterest in and lack of involvement in what appeared to be an active and engaging classroom. On questioning, parents and teachers indicated that they had considered depression might be a component of the problem but had assumed that the girl's somber mood was reflective of school difficulties and the pressure she felt to perform. An informal academic survey revealed fair reading ability, a distaste for math, and some problems with written production. An interview with the young woman indicated moderate depression during at least the last 6-month period, currently exacerbated by a disruption in family relationships and rejection by a key peer in the classroom, as well as some long-standing discomfort with school. Further evaluation by a learning disabilities specialist revealed specific skill deficits in writing and math. Initial intervention began with counseling and medication for the depression, a resolution of the teasing by the peer, and some individual help in writing and math. In the early stages, executive skill weaknesses were managed by external support from teaching staff with no emphasis on the young woman learning and internalizing these skills until she showed definite progress with the depression and academic weaknesses. Thus, a case that initially and reasonably appeared to be a set of problems related to executive skill deficits turned out, on further examination, to involve a more complex set of issues. In situations such as this where the initial presumption is one of executive skill weaknesses, certain findings might signal otherwise. Hence, it is important to understand that presenting problems such as decreased work output, missing deadlines, and losing materials can be influenced by variables other than or in addition to executive skills. Understanding what these variables are and the symptoms/behaviors by which they are manifest is critical to an accurate assessment and to an effective intervention. While in such cases a full evaluation may not be necessary, sufficient information needs to be gathered through observation, record review, checklists, and interviews to rule out learning, emotional, and psychosocial issues as principle factors or causes.

Complicated cases involving executive skills can also present at the outset as just that—complicated cases. Thus, children can be referred with evidence or a strong suspicion of cognitive/learning disabilities, attention disorders, and/or emotional/social problems. If no or only limited assessment has been completed prior to referral, an evaluation sufficiently comprehensive to document functioning in these areas should be completed. Assessment of executive skills should be one component. The intended outcome of this comprehensive evaluation is a detailed, integrated picture of the child's strengths and weaknesses in these different areas and how they contribute to the level of functioning and to the referral issue. For children beyond the early grades, evaluations often have been completed. In this case, rather than a comprehensive evaluation, the objective is to gather existing information, supplement for any missing evaluation pieces, and develop the same integrated picture. In either circumstance, children who manifest with complex problems (e.g., learning disabilities or emotional disorders) are already at risk for school failure. Executive skill weaknesses can compound the risk because of the role they play in work production and because as the child matures, there are fewer naturally occurring supports for these skill in the environment. Hence, it is important to assess these skills even when other significant problems have been identified. If executive weaknesses are identified, it is important to explain how these weaknesses interact with other problems, how they are likely to impact performance now and in future, and what types of support the student will need currently and in the coming grades to manage increasing demands.

CONCLUDING COMMENTS

To aid the reader in understanding the complex process of designing and implementing interventions to address executive skill deficits, we would like to reiterate some points we've alluded to before and make some observations on the processes involved in helping children improve executive skills. These are things we believe parents and teachers need to be particularly mindful of as they embark on their efforts to teach executive skills.

- It is important to keep a developmental perspective in mind when making decisions about remediating executive skill deficits. Younger children in general have weak executive skills. Parents and teachers make up for these weaknesses by imposing structure and providing massive environmental supports. As a first step for children with weak executive skills, we encourage those who work with them to make sure environmental supports are in place before beginning to teach children to use executive skills on their own. Teachers in particular need to be mindful of what children at different ages are capable of. Remember: it takes nearly *two decades* for frontal lobes to reach maturation. In particular, we believe that the jump in expectations for independent functioning that occurs when students begin middle school often is likely to be inconsistent with children's developmental capabilities. And we urge teachers at all levels to resist ramping up expectations for students "to prepare them for the next grade level." Often, this simply increases the mismatch between expectations for child behavior and developmental readiness.

- Keep in mind that executive skills, like all cognitive and psychological traits, fall along a continuum. Children can be very poor at sustaining attention or initiating tasks, or they can have mild problems, or they can be very good at them. Parents and teachers need to recognize the severity of the problem in the individual children they work with and adjust their efforts accordingly. In many cases, problems will require a long-term improvement plan.

- Our manual has not addressed directly the problem of the resistant child. It assumes, rather, that youngsters are open to the idea of working on improving executive functioning. If this is not the case, then beginning with a motivational component such as a reward or incentive system may be the place to start. Even with this intervention, however, we expect there will be youngsters who continue to be highly resistant to efforts to improve executive skills. When this is encountered, an assessment is recommended to help understand the nature and cause of the resistance. This may be either a functional behavioral assessment or a more traditional psychological assessment. It may be that progress is impeded by other, unidentified learning problems or processing disorders, or it may reside in family dynamics, to name just a few possible factors that may need to be considered.

• Even under optimal conditions (able teachers, willing children, well-designed interventions), we caution against expecting students to show quick improvement. These are skills that take time to develop. We frequently say to both parents and teachers that progress is better measured in years than in months. But even if progress is not readily apparent as fast as would be desired, do not give up on teaching these procedures. Children *can* incorporate them over time, and they will learn skills that are critical to success in high school and college and on into adulthood.

• Use a combination of interventions—environmental modifications, incentive systems, and strategy training—and don't move too quickly to drop environmental modifications or incentives. If you do move too quickly and the process begins to unravel, slow it down by putting back environmental supports or beefing up incentives.

• At the same time, adults need to know when to ease up the supports and cuing in order for children to develop more independence. Keep in mind that by the time youngsters graduate from high school, they are expected to function independently. Ideally, this means that they have fully functioning frontal lobes that manage their ability to execute tasks of daily living. This is particularly true of youngsters going on to college, since the demands on time management, planning/organization, and goal-directed persistence in this setting are particularly pronounced. Those who work with youngsters with executive skill deficits should set as their goal that no later than midway through their senior year these students can function successfully with minimal or no cues or supports from adults other than those that naturally occur in their environment. If they are not functioning successfully on their own, it will be important to plan for how these issues will be addressed in college.

• When working with children with more pervasive deficits, do not try to teach too many skills all at once. Rather, identify those skills that are most critical for school success over time and focus on these. Trying to tackle too many skills is not only difficult to achieve but also may result in both the child and others as seeing him as a child with many deficits rather than a child with lots of talents and potential. It helps both to keep the "big picture" in mind (what's *really* important) and to take a long-term view of the problem (i.e., the skills we want the child to have by the time he finishes high school).

• Make the purpose of instruction explicit. Tell the child, "Here's what we're working on and here's why." This both increases the likelihood that the child will "get it" and that she can use her own problem-solving skills to address difficult areas. This will not only give the child more ownership over problems and more motivation to solve them, but it also means her knowledge of herself and her problem-solving skills can be harnessed to generate good solutions.

• Well functioning executive skills are defined by *self*-regulation of behavior. Hence, the active participation of the child in planning and implementation of strategies is an essential component of successful intervention. When the child is not involved, the goal of intervention—the development of executive skills—is not met. On the other hand, when the child is involved, the very act of participation enhances skills such as planning and metacognition and enhances the child's sense of self-regulation. In addition, when the child chooses strategies, goodness of fit with current skills is more likely, as is the actual use of the strategies. There also is increasing evidence in the educational and psychological literature indicating that students who play an active role in planning and decision making relevant to their education perform better than do peers who are not involved (Field & Hoffman, 2002). For these reasons we believe that children should be encouraged to participate in developing interventions for executive skills at whatever level is appropriate for their age and level of cognitive development.

• Teaching executive skills is labor intensive. As we noted in Chapter 4, we encourage teachers to think about ways they can use group instruction to teach critical executive skills. While some students may not need this kind of lesson, we believe that many if not most students would gain from explicit instruction, especially if it incorporates a problem-solving process where students can be called on to help each other develop more effective executive skills.

Finally, we have included an Appendix with a variety of forms and checklists that can be used to assess executive skills and assist in developing interventions. While some of these may be used as given, we encourage readers to see them as models that can be adapted to fit the unique circumstances of the children with whom they are working.

We have attempted in this manual to tell the reader everything we know about executive skills. Well, not everything, because our knowledge of these skills and how they develop in children keeps evolving. We are convinced, however—and this is unlikely to change—that if executive skills are taught explicitly by parents and teachers, then children not only will become more effective students but will acquire a set of skills that contribute to adult success both in the home and in the workplace. This was brought home to us recently when we conducted a workshop for teachers on executive skills. We began by presenting our model and asking them to think about ways they use executive skills in their daily teaching practice. "Is there any one of these skills you don't use to be an effective teacher?" we asked. The consensus of the group was that each skill was essential. And teaching, clearly, is not the only profession where strong executive skills are critical.

Appendix

EXECUTIVE SKILLS SEMISTRUCTURED INTERVIEW—PARENT VERSION

Many youngsters have problems in school or with homework not because they lack intelligence but because they have weak executive skills. These refer to the skills required to plan/prioritize (P) and carry out tasks, including time management (TM), working memory (WM), the ability to organize tasks and materials (O), task initiation (TI) and follow-through, flexibility (F), response inhibition (RI), self-regulation of affect (SRA), sustained attention (SA), goal-directed persistence (GDP), and metacognition (M). I'm going to ask you some questions about _____ (fill in the child's name) to help us get a clearer understanding of his or her executive skills. Codes in parentheses refer to the specific executive skill measured by each item.

HOMEWORK. Which of the following areas, if any, does your child have difficulty with?

Item	Notes
Understanding homework directions (M)	
Getting started on his own (TI)	
Being able to keep working despite distractions (SA)	
Asking for help when it's needed (M)	
Sticking with it long enough to complete it (SA, GDP)	
Making careless mistakes; failing to check work (M)	
Finishing the work on time (TM)	
Remembering to hand it in (WM)	

Are there some subjects or kinds of assignments your child is more likely than others to complete successfully?

More likely to be successful with . . .	Less likely to be successful with . . .

(continued)

ORGANIZATION OF MATERIALS. Which of the following areas does your child have difficulty with?

Item	Notes
Keeping notebooks and papers organized (O)	
Keeping desk tidy (O)	
Keeping belongings neat and in appropriate locations (e.g., gym clothes, coats, hats, mittens) (O)	
Keeping track of books, papers, pencils, etc. (O)	
Keeping knapsack organized (O)	

LONG-TERM PROJECTS. Which of the following areas does your child have difficulty with?

Item	Notes
Deciding on a topic (P)	
Breaking the assignment into smaller parts (P)	
Developing a timeline (P)	
Following a timeline (TM)	
Estimating how long it will take to finish (TM)	
Following directions carefully (WM, M)	
Proofreading or checking project to catch mistakes to make sure the rules were followed (M)	
Finishing the project by the deadline (GDP)	

(continued)

REMEMBERING. Which of the following areas does your child have difficulty with?

Item	Notes
Writing down assignments (WM)	
Bringing home appropriate materials (e.g., books, workbooks, assignment book, worksheets, notices, permission slips, gym clothes) (WM)	
Bringing to school appropriate materials (see examples above) (WM)	
Remembering instructional sequences after normal instruction (e.g., long division, proper headings for papers) (WM)	
Remembering to perform chores or other household responsibilities (WM)	
Losing things within the home, yard, or neighborhood (WM)	

PROBLEM SOLVING. Which of the following areas does your child have difficulty with?

Item	Notes
Recognizing that he or she has a problem (e.g., doesn't understand the directions) (M)	
Being able to think flexibly about the problem (i.e., not get stuck on one approach, solution, etc.) (F)	
Trying to solve the problem first on his or her own before going for help (M)	
Accessing appropriate resources to help him or her solve the problem (F)	
Evaluating his or her own performance to know whether the problem was solved successfully (M)	

(continued)

SELF-CONTROL. Some youngsters have difficulty managing their behavior. Which of the following areas does your child have difficulty with?

Item	Notes
Becoming easily upset (SRA)	
Throwing temper tantrums (SRA)	
Acting impulsively, either verbally or physically (e.g., provoking siblings) (RI)	
Interrupting others (RI)	
Difficulty waiting turn (RI)	

PARENTAL EXECUTIVE SKILLS. Do you see yourself as having challenges in any of the areas we've talked about? If so, in which areas?

Can you envision other problems with starting or following a plan? How or by whom could these problems be managed?

EXECUTIVE SKILLS SEMISTRUCTURED INTERVIEW—TEACHER VERSION

Many youngsters have problems in school or with homework not because they lack intelligence but because they have weak executive skills. These refer to the skills required to plan/prioritize (P) and carry out tasks, including time management (TM), working memory (WM), the ability to organize tasks and materials (O), task initiation (TI) and follow-through, flexibility (F), response inhibition (RI), self-regulation of affect (SRA), sustained attention (SA), goal-directed persistence (GDP), and metacognition (M). I'm going to ask you some questions about _____ (fill in the child's name) to help us get a clearer understanding of his or her executive skills. Codes in parentheses refer to the specific executive skill measured by each item.

INDEPENDENT SEATWORK. Which of the following areas, if any, does the student have difficulty with?

Item	Notes
Understanding task directions (M)	
Getting started on his own (TI)	
Being able to keep working despite distractions (SA)	
Asking for help when it's needed (M)	
Sticking with it long enough to complete it (SA, GDP)	
Making careless mistakes; failing to check work (M)	
Finishing the work on time (TM)	
Remembering to hand it in (WM)	

Are there some subjects or kinds of assignments which the student is more likely than others to complete successfully?

More likely to be successful with . . .	Less likely to be successful with . . .

(continued)

ORGANIZATION OF MATERIALS. Which of the following areas does the student have difficulty with?

Item	Notes
Keeping notebooks and papers organized (O)	
Keeping desk tidy (O)	
Keeping belongings neat and in appropriate locations (e.g., gym clothes, coats, hats, mittens) (O)	
Keeping track of books, papers, pencils, etc. (O)	
Keeping knapsack organized (O)	

LONG-TERM PROJECTS. Which of the following areas does the student have difficulty with?

Item	Notes
Deciding on a topic (P)	
Breaking the assignment into smaller parts (P)	
Developing a timeline (P)	
Following a timeline (TM)	
Estimating how long it will take to finish (TM)	
Following directions carefully (WM, M)	
Proofreading or checking project to catch mistakes to make sure the rules were followed (M)	
Finishing the project by the deadline (GDP)	

(continued)

REMEMBERING. Which of the following areas does the student have difficulty with?

Item	Notes
Writing down assignments (WM)	
Bringing home appropriate materials (e.g., books, workbooks, assignment book, worksheets, notices, permission slips, gym clothes) (WM)	
Bringing to school appropriate materials (see examples above) (WM)	
Remembering to follow classroom procedures (WM)	
Losing things in the classroom or other places in the school (e.g., lunchroom, gym, playground) (WM)	
Remembering instructional sequences after normal instruction (e.g., long division, proper headings for papers) (WM)	

PROBLEM SOLVING. Which of the following areas does the student have difficulty with?

Item	Notes
Recognizing that he or she has a problem (e.g., doesn't understand the directions) (M)	
Being able to think flexibly about the problem (i.e., not get stuck on one approach, solution, etc.) (F)	
Trying to solve the problem first on his or her own before going for help (M)	
Accessing appropriate resources to help him or her solve the problem (F)	
Evaluating his or her own performance to know whether the problem was solved successfully (M)	

(continued)

SELF-CONTROL. Some youngsters have difficulty managing their behavior. Which of the following areas does the student have difficulty with?

Item	Notes
Becoming easily upset (SRA)	
Throwing temper tantrums (SRA)	
Acting impulsively, either verbally or physically (e.g., provoking siblings) (RI)	
Interrupting others (RI)	
Difficulty waiting turn (RI)	

CURRENT EFFORTS TO ADDRESS THE PROBLEM. Please identify the current strategies or interventions that are being used to address this student's problem areas and indicate how successful they are.

TEACHER EXECUTIVE SKILLS. Do you consider yourself as having challenges in any of the areas we've talked about? If so, will this have an impact on your ability to put in place interventions to address the student's problem areas?

EXECUTIVE SKILLS SEMISTRUCTURED INTERVIEW—STUDENT VERSION

I'm going to ask you some questions about situations related to your success as a student. All of these are situations in which you have to use planning and organizational skills in order to be successful. Some will be directly related to school, whereas other questions will touch on extracurricular activities, any job situations you've been in, and how you spend your leisure time.

HOMEWORK. I'm going to ask you some questions about homework and the kinds of problems kids sometimes have with homework. Please tell me if you think these are problems for you. I may ask you to give me examples of how you see it as a problem.

Item	Notes
Getting started on homework. (TI) *Related questions:* What makes it hard? When is the best time to do homework? Are some subjects harder to start than others?	
Sticking with it long enough to get it done. (SA) *Related questions:* Is this worse with some subjects than others? What do you say to yourself that either leads you to give up or stick with it? Does the length of the assignment make a difference in your ability to complete it?	
Remembering assignments. (WM) *Related questions:* Do you have trouble remembering to write down assignments, bring home necessary materials, or hand in assignments? Do you lose things necessary to complete the task?	
Becoming distracted while doing homework. (SA) *Related questions:* What kinds of things distract you? Have you found places to study that minimize distractions? How do you handle the distractions when they come up?	
Having other things you'd rather do. (P, GDP) *Related questions:* Are there things you have trouble tearing yourself away from to do homework? Do you resent having homework or too much homework? Do you think there are other things in your life that are more important than homework?	

(continued)

LONG-TERM PROJECTS. Now let's talk about long-term assignments. Which of the following are hard for you?

Item	Notes
Choosing a topic (M)	
Breaking the assignment into smaller parts (P)	
Developing a timeline (P)	
Sticking with a timeline (TM)	
Estimating how long it will take to finish (TM)	
Following directions (e.g., do you forget to do part of the assignment and lose points as a result?) (WM, M)	
Proofreading or checking your work to make sure you followed the rules and haven't made careless mistakes (M)	
Finishing the project by the deadline (GDP)	

STUDYING FOR TESTS. Here are some problems students sometimes have when studying for tests. Which ones are a problem for you?

Item	Notes
Making yourself sit down and study (TI)	
Knowing what to study (M)	
Knowing how to study (M)	
Putting off studying/not studying at all (TM)	

(continued)

STUDYING FOR TESTS. *(continued)*

Taking breaks that are either too frequent or too long (SA)	
Giving up before you've studied enough (GDP)	
Memorizing the material (WM)	
Understanding the material (M)	

HOME CHORES/RESPONSIBILITIES. What kinds of chores do you have to do on a regular or irregular basis?

Chore	Regular (When do you do it?)	Occasional
1.		
2.		
3.		
4.		
5.		

What aspects of completing chores do you have trouble with?

Item	Notes
Remembering to do them (WM)	
Doing them when you're supposed to (TI)	
Running out of steam before you're done (SA)	
Doing a sloppy job and getting in trouble for it (M)	

(continued)

ORGANIZATIONAL SKILLS. Now I'm going to ask some questions about how organized you are. Tell me if you have problems with any of the following.

Item	Notes
Keeping your bedroom neat (O)	
Keeping your notebooks organized (O)	
Keeping your knapsack organized (O)	
Keeping your desk clean (O)	
Keeping your locker clean (O)	
Leaving your belongings all over the house (O)	
Leaving belongings other places (e.g., school, friend's houses, at work) (O)	
Losing or misplacing things (O)	

WORK/LEISURE TIME. Let's talk about how you spend your time when you're not in school. What kinds of extracurricular activities are you involved in? Do you have a job? How do you spend your leisure time?

Activity	Amount of time (approximate per day or week)
1.	
2.	
3.	
4.	
5.	
6.	
7.	

(continued)

Here are some problems that students sometimes have with how they spend their spare time. Which ones are problems for you?

Item	Notes
Spending too many hours at a job (TM)	
"Wasting" time (e.g., hanging out, playing computer/ video games, talking on the phone, going on the Internet, watching too much TV) (TM)	
Hanging out with kids who get in trouble (RI)	
Not getting enough sleep (RI)	
Spending money as soon as you get it (RI)	

LONG-TERM GOALS. Do you know what you want to do after high school?

Possible goals
1.
2.
3.
4.

Have you formulated a plan for reaching your goal(s)? If so, what is it?

(continued)

What are some of the potential obstacles that might prevent you from reaching your goal?

Potential obstacle	Ways to overcome the obstacle
1.	
2.	
3.	
4.	
5.	

If you have not yet identified a goal or developed a plan for reaching the goal, when do you think you will you do this?

EXECUTIVE SKILLS: PLANNING INTERVENTIONS

Student Name: _____   Date: _____

I. Data Sources—check all that apply

_____ Parent Interview	_____ Parent Checklists	_____ Classroom Observation
_____ Teacher Interview	_____ Teacher Checklists	_____ Work Samples
_____ Student Interview	_____ Student Checklists	_____ Formal Assessment

II. Areas of Need—fill in applicable sections

Response Inhibition (RI): The capacity to think before acting

Specific problem behaviors (e.g., talks out in class; interrupts; says things without thinking)
1.
2.
3.

Working Memory (WM): The ability to hold information in memory while performing complex tasks

Specific problem behaviors (e.g., forgets directions; leaves homework at home; can't do mental arithmetic)
1.
2.
3.

Self-Regulation of Affect (SRA): The ability to manage emotions in order to achieve goals, complete tasks, or control or direct behavior

Specific problem behaviors (e.g., "freezes" on tests; gets frustrated when makes mistakes; stops trying in the face of challenge)
1.
2.
3.

Sustained Attention (SA): The capacity to maintain attention to a situation or task in spite of distractibility, fatigue, or boredom

Specific problem behaviors (e.g., fails to complete classwork on time; stops work before finishing)
1.
2.
3.

(continued)

Task Initiation (TI): The ability to begin projects without undue procrastination, in an efficient or timely fashion

Specific problem behaviors (e.g., needs cues to start work; puts off long-term assignments)

   1.

   2.

   3.

Planning/Prioritization (P): The ability to create a roadmap to reach a goal or to complete a task

Specific problem behaviors (e.g., doesn't know where to start an assignment; can't develop a timeline for long-term assignments)

   1.

   2.

   3.

Organization (O): The ability to arrange or place things according to a system

Specific problem behaviors (e.g., doesn't write down assignments; loses books or papers)

   1.

   2.

   3.

Time Management (TM): The capacity to estimate how much time one has, how to allocate it, and how to stay within time limits and deadlines

Specific problem behaviors (e.g., doesn't work efficiently; can't estimate how long it takes to do something)

   1.

   2.

   3.

Goal-Directed Persistence (GDP): The capacity to have a goal, follow through to the completion of the goal, and not be put off by or distracted by competing interests

Specific problem behaviors (e.g., doesn't see connection between homework and long-term goals; doesn't follow through to achieve stated goals)

   1.

   2.

   3.

Flexibility (F): The ability to revise plans in the face of obstacles, setbacks, new information, or mistakes; it relates to an adaptability to changing conditions

Specific problem behaviors (e.g., gets stuck on one problem-solving strategy; gets upset by unexpected changes to schedule or plans)

   1.

   2.

   3.

(continued)

Metacognition (M): The ability to stand back and take a bird's-eye view of oneself in a situation; the ability to self-monitor and self-evaluate

Specific problem behaviors (e.g., doesn't have effective study strategies; difficulty catching or correcting mistakes)

   1.

   2.

   3.

III. Establish Goal Behavior—select specific skill to work on

Target Executive Skill: _____

Specific Behavioral Objective: _____

_____

IV. Design Intervention

What environmental supports or modifications will be provided to help reach the target goal?

What specific skills will be taught, who will teach skill, and what procedure will be used to teach the skill(s)?

Skill:

Who will teach skill:

Procedure:

(continued)

Skill:

Who will teach skill:

Procedure:

What incentives will be used to help motivate the student to use/practice the skill(s)?

V. Evaluate Intervention

Review date: _____

Was the behavioral objective met?   Yes, completely _____   Yes, partially _____   No _____

Assessment of efficacy of intervention components:

Environmental Supports/Modifications
Were they put in place?
Were they effective?
Do they need to be continued?
Plan for fading supports:

(continued)

Skill Instruction
Was the instruction implemented?
What was the outcome?
Does the instruction need to be continued?
Plan for fading instruction:

Incentives
Were incentives used?
Were they effective?
Do they need to be continued?
Plan for fading incentives:

Date for next review: _____

INCENTIVE PLANNING SHEET

Problem Behavior

Goal

Possible Rewards

| Daily | Weekly | Long-Term |

Possible Contingencies

BEHAVIOR CONTRACT

Student agrees to _____

_____

To help student reach goal, parents will _____

_____

Student will earn _____

_____

If student fails to meet agreement, student will _____

_____

HOMEWORK CHECKLIST

Date: _____

Tasks	Yes	No
All assignments written in assignment book		
All necessary books/papers in knapsack to go home: Check off below. _____ English _____ Social Studies _____ Math _____ Reading _____ Science _____ Spelling _____ Other:		
Other things to go home: Check off below. _____ Permission slips _____ Clothing _____ Notices _____ Sports equipment _____ Teacher notes _____ Other:		
All homework completed: Check off below. _____ English _____ Social Studies _____ Math _____ Reading _____ Science _____ Spelling _____ Other:		
Homework placed in appropriate folders		
Homework folders in knapsack		
Other things to go to school: Check off below. _____ Permission slips _____ Clothing _____ Notices _____ Sports equipment _____ Notes to teacher _____ Lunch money or lunch		
All homework handed in to teacher: Check off below. _____ English _____ Social Studies _____ Math _____ Reading _____ Science _____ Spelling _____ Other:		

LONG-TERM PROJECT PLANNING SHEET

STEP 1: SELECT TOPIC

What are possible topics?	What I like about this choice:	What I don't like:
1.		
2.		
3.		
4.		
5.		

Final Topic Choice:

STEP 2: IDENTIFY NECESSARY MATERIALS

What materials or resources do you need?	Where will you get them?	When will you get them?
1.		
2.		
3.		
4.		
5.		

(continued)

STEP 3: IDENTIFY PROJECT TASKS AND DUE DATES

What do you need to do? (List each step in order.)	When will you do it?	Check off when done
Step 1:		
Step 2:		
Step 3:		
Step 4:		
Step 5:		
Step 6:		
Step 7:		
Step 8:		
Step 9:		
Step 10:		

HOMEWORK PLANNING SHEET

Date: _____

Subject 1: _____

Assignment: _____

_____

_____

What materials do I need?

_____ Worksheet   _____ Writing Materials

_____ Textbook   _____ Calculator

_____ Workbook   _____ Computer

_____ Other (describe):

How long will it take me to complete this assignment?_____

When do I plan to start? _____

ACTUAL START TIME: _____

TIME TASK COMPLETED: _____

Subject 2: _____

Assignment: _____

_____

_____

_____

What materials do I need?

____ Worksheet   ____ Writing materials

____ Textbook   ____ Calculator

____ Workbook   ____ Computer

____ Other (describe):

How long will it take me to complete this assignment? _____

When do I plan to start? _____

ACTUAL START TIME: _____

TIME TASK COMPLETED: _____

DESK CLEANING CHECKLIST

STEP 1: GATHER NECESSARY MATERIALS

Materials needed	Check all that apply
Wastebasket	
Empty file folders	
Three-ring binders	
Paper clips	
Stapler	
Manila envelopes	

STEP 2: FOLLOW DESK-CLEANING PROCEDURE

Procedure	Check when done
Empty out desk	
Sort everything into two piles: *Save/Don't Save*	
Throw *Don't Save* pile in wastebasket	
Sort *Save* pile into two piles: 1. School stuff (books, unfinished assignments, assignments that are completed but the teacher wants me to save, pens, pencils, etc.) 2. Home stuff (notices/slips to give parents, assignments I want to save but don't have to keep for teacher, uneaten snacks, etc.)	
Put "home stuff" in knapsack to go home (in folders or manila envelopes if necessary)	
Sort "school stuff": one pile for each subject, one extra pile for "other"	
Organize each subject pile following teacher instructions (e.g., placing materials by date in three-ring binders or folders)	
Decide what to do with the "other" pile	
Put all school materials neatly back in desk	

CHORE PLANNING SHEET

Date: _____   Chore: _____

What materials do I need?

What steps do I need to follow to complete this chore?	Check when completed
1.	
2.	
3.	
4.	
5.	
6.	

Will I need help completing this chore? (Circle one)   YES   NO

If I need help, who will help me? _____

How long will it take me to do this chore?_____

When do I plan to start? _____

ACTUAL START TIME: _____

TIME TASK COMPLETED: _____

CHANGING CLASSES

Class: _____

Steps to follow	Check when done
Hand in yesterday's assignments.	
Write down homework for tonight.	
Have all necessary materials in knapsack. • Assignment book • Textbook • Notebook • Worksheet • Pencils/pens	
Check around desk/class for other belongings (clothes, gym clothes, etc.).	

Class: _____

Steps to follow	Check when done
Hand in yesterday's assignments.	
Write down homework for tonight.	
Have all necessary materials in knapsack. • Assignment book • Textbook • Notebook • Worksheet • Pencils/pens	
Check around desk/class for other belongings (clothes, gym clothes, etc.).	

CLASSWORK PLANNING SHEET

Date: _____

Assignment: _____

_____

_____

What materials do I need?

____ Worksheet   ____ Writing materials

____ Textbook   ____ Calculator

____ Workbook   ____ Computer

____ Other (describe):

How long will it take me to complete this assignment?_____

What do I need to do in order to stay focused on this task? (e.g., sit away from distractions, don't talk to classmates, remind myself "Get back to work," tell myself I'm doing a good job staying on task, etc.)

When do I plan to start? _____

ACTUAL START TIME: _____

TIME TASK COMPLETED:_____

How did I do? Circle one:

Great!   Pretty good   Could have done better   Had a hard time today

What could I do differently the next time to be more successful?

GETTING READY TO GO HOME

Steps to follow	Check when done
Hand in any homework assignments completed.	
Hand in any in-class assignments completed.	
Return any materials borrowed from classmates or teacher.	
Tidy up desk surface; check floor around desk.	
Gather all necessary materials to go home:	
1. Books	
2. Notebooks	
3. Folders	
4. Assignment book	
5. Worksheets	
6. Slips/notices for parents	
7. Clothing (hat, mittens, coat)	
8. Gym clothes	
9. Other:	
Place appropriate materials in knapsack.	
Ask myself, Am I forgetting anything?	

DAILY HOMEWORK PLANNER

Date: _____

Subject/Assignment	Do I have all the materials?	Do I need help?	Who will help me?	How long will it take?	When will I start?
	Yes ☐ No ☐	Yes ☐ No ☐			
	Yes ☐ No ☐	Yes ☐ No ☐			
	Yes ☐ No ☐	Yes ☐ No ☐			
	Yes ☐ No ☐	Yes ☐ No ☐			
	Yes ☐ No ☐	Yes ☐ No ☐			
	Yes ☐ No ☐	Yes ☐ No ☐			

When will I take breaks?	What will be my reward for following my plan?

References

Achenbach, T. M. (1991a). *Child Behavior Checklist*. Burlington: University of Vermont.

Achenbach, T. M. (1991b). *Child Behavior Checklist—Teacher Report Form*. Burlington: University of Vermont.

Alberto, P. A., & Troutman, A. C. (1999). *Applied behavior analysis for teachers* (5th ed.). Upper Saddler River, NJ: Prentice-Hall.

Barkley, R. A. (1997). *ADHD and the nature of self-control*. New York: Guilford Press.

Bronson, M. B. (2000). *Self-regulation in early childhood*. New York: Guilford Press.

Conners, K. (2000). *Conners' Continuous Performance Test—II*. North Tonawanda, NY: Multi-Health Systems.

Dahl, R. E. (1999). In K. L. Wahlstrom (Ed.), *Adolescent sleep needs and school starting times* (pp. 29–34). Bloomington, IN: Phi Delta Kappa Educational Foundation.

Dawson, P., & Guare, R. (1998). *Coaching the ADHD student*. North Tonawanda, NY: Multi-Health Systems.

Delis, D., Kaplan, E., & Kramer, J. (2000). *Delis–Kaplan Executive Function Scale*. San Antonio, TX: Psychological Corporation.

DuPaul, G. J., Power, T. J., Anastopoulos, A. D., & Reid, R. (1998). *ADHD Rating Scale—IV*. New York: Guilford Press.

Field, S., & Hoffman, A. (2002). Lessons learned from implementing the *Steps to Self-Determination* curriculum. *Remedial and Special Education, 23,* 90–98.

Frey, W. F. (1994). Psychotherapeutic interventions for mild traumatic brain injury. In R. C. Savage & G. F. Wolcott (Eds.), *Educational dimensions of acquired brain injury* (pp. 319–341). Austin, TX: PRO-ED.

Gioia, G. A., Isquith, P. K., Guy, S. C., & Kenworthy, L. (2000). *Behavior Rating Inventory of Executive Function*. Odessa, FL: Psychological Assessment Resources.

Hallowell, E., & Ratey, J. (1994). *Driven to distraction*. New York: Pantheon.

Hart, T., & Jacobs, H. E. (1993). Rehabilitation and management of behavioral disturbances following frontal lobe injury. *Journal of Head Trauma Rehabilitation, 8,* 1–12.

Heaton, R. K. (1981). *Wisconsin Card Sorting Test (WCST)*. Odessa, FL: Psychological Assessment Resources.

Kagan, J. (1966). Reflection-impulsivity: The generality and dynamics of conceptual tempo. *Journal of Abnormal Psychology, 71,* 17–24.

Kolb, B., & Wishaw, Q. (1990). *Fundamentals of neuropsychology* (3rd ed.). New York: Freeman.

Korkman, M., Kirk, U., & Kemp, S. (1998). *NEPSY.* San Antonio, TX: Psychological Corporation.

Mesulam, M.-M. (1985). *Principles of behavioral neurology.* Philadelphia: Davis.

Naglieri, J., & Das, J. P. (1997). *Cognitive Assessment System.* Itasca, IL: Riverside.

National Sleep Foundation. (1999). *Omnibus sleep in America poll.* Washington, DC: Author.

Neeper, R., Lahey, B. B., & Frick, P. A. (1990) *Comprehensive Behavior Rating Scale for Children.* San Antonio, TX: Psychological Corporation.

Ozonoff, S., & Griffith, E. M. (2000). Neuropsychological function and the external validity of Asperger Syndrome. In A. Klin, F. R. Volkmar, & S. S. Sparrow (Eds.), *Asperger syndrome* (pp. 72–96). New York: Guilford Press.

Paniagua, F. A. (1992). Verbal–nonverbal correspondence training with ADHD children. *Behavior Modification, 16,* 226–252.

Pelayo, R. P., Thorpy, M. J., & Glovinsky, P. (1988). Prevalence of delayed sleep phase syndrome among adolescents. *Sleep Research, 17,* 391.

Pliszka, S. R. (2002). Neuroimaging and ADHD: Recent progress. *The ADHD Report, 10*(3), 1–6.

Porteus, S. D. (1959). *The Maze Test and clinical psychology.* Palo Alto, CA: Pacific Books.

Reitan, R. M., & Wolfson, D. (1985). *The Halstead–Reitan Neuropsychological Test Battery.* Tucson, AZ: Neuropsychological Press.

Rourke, B. P., & Tsatsanis, K. D. (2000). Nonverbal learning disabilities and Asperger syndrome. In A. Klin, F. R. Volkmar, & S. S. Sparrow (Eds.), *Asperger syndrome* (pp. 231–253). New York: Guilford Press.

Savage, R. C., & Wolcott, G. F. (1994). Overview of acquired brain injury. In R. C. Savage & G. F. Wolcott (Eds.), *Educational dimensions of acquired brain injury* (pp. 3–12). Austin, TX: PRO-ED.

Sheslow, D., & Adams, W. (1990). *Wide Range Assessment of Memory and Learning.* Wilmington, DE: Wide Range.

Wahlstrom, K. A. (Ed.). (1999). *Adolescent sleep needs and school starting times.* Bloomington, IN: Phi Delta Kappa Educational Foundation.

Wechsler, D. (1991). *Wechsler Intelligence Scale for Children—Third Edition.* San Antonio, TX: Psychological Corporation.

Ylvisaker, M., Szekeres, S. F., & Hartwick, P. (1994). A framework for cognitive intervention. In R. C. Savage & G. F. Wolcott (Eds.), *Educational dimensions of acquired brain injury* (pp. 35–67). Austin, TX: PRO-ED.

Index